Advancing Global Bioethics

Volume 17

The book series Global Bioethics provides a forum for normative analysis of a vast range of important new issues in bioethics from a truly global perspective and with a cross-cultural approach. The issues covered by the series include among other things sponsorship of research and education, scientific misconduct and research integrity, exploitation of research participants in resource-poor settings, brain drain and migration of healthcare workers, organ trafficking and transplant tourism, indigenous medicine, biodiversity, commodification of human tissue, benefit sharing, bio-industry and food, malnutrition and hunger, human rights, and climate change.

More information about this series at https://link.springer.com/bookseries/10420

Pierre Mallia • Nathan Emmerich
Bert Gordijn • Francesca Pistoia
Editors

Challenges to the Global Issue of End of Life Care

Training and Implementing Change

Springer

Editors
Pierre Mallia
Medical School
University of Malta
Msida, Malta

Bert Gordijn
Institute of Ethics
Dublin City University
Dublin, Ireland

Nathan Emmerich
Australian National University
Canberra, Australia

Francesca Pistoia
Neurological Institute
University of L'Aquila
Coppito, L'Aquila, Italy

ISSN 2212-652X ISSN 2212-6538 (electronic)
Advancing Global Bioethics
ISBN 978-3-030-86385-2 ISBN 978-3-030-86386-9 (eBook)
https://doi.org/10.1007/978-3-030-86386-9

This Springer imprint is published by the registered company Springer Nature Switzerland AG
The registered company address is: Gewerbestrasse 11, 6330 Cham, Switzerland

This book is dedicated to our family and friends who have given their support and to those who care for the dying patient

Preface

End of Life (EoL) care is a field which attracts global attention and which, notwithstanding moral agreement on most issues contextually, continues globally to be a source of controversy. The reasons vary between countries from lack of clarity about law, lack of health professionals and the public on accepted moral norms, and difficulty to implement change contextually. The amount of literature and popular books published by experienced help professionals showing their frustrations in the field is testament to the medicalisation of end of life care in hospital. Whilst many religions and philosophy agree on the exception of extraordinary or futile treatment as passive euthanasia and that pain relief ought not to be considered in any way as active hastening of a terminally ill patient, comparative studies do show that in many cultures and religions this continues to be problem globally with many health professionals and patients (including their relatives) not knowing the issues well. Conversely, whilst in many countries there seems to be an increase in the number of patients who request euthanasia, as well as arguments for its legalisation based on the patients' right to make autonomous choices, some research shows that these requests may result from an improper implementation of EoL care. Many people feel they should not die in pain unnecessarily, nor do they want to be hooked up to machines. They do not seem to realise that pain relief, even if it risks hastening death, and the refusal of treatment are recognised moral rights.

In fact, euthanasia aside, end of life care is probably the less controversial field apart from arguments such as what constitutes 'futile' treatment. Problems are more inherent in systems and in lack of understanding or due to the emotional charge of situations.

Tackling these problems is the subject of this book. There is a sea between theoretical bioethics, which gives us the necessary grounding of our moral actions, and clinical ethics when one is faced with a real patient and real relatives, and not least a team which not only wants to do well by the patient but wants to be seen to be doing what is just. All hospitals face problems with communication, with advanced care planning, with talking to patients and relatives and even inter- and intra-professional communication and agreement. Many of course do not come from a philosophical background and would not understand the moral equivalence principle between omitting to start treatment and withdrawing treatment which is being given, the latter being seen more emotionally charged. This shows that end of life is not merely a philosophical problem but goes in the realm of psychosocial issues. This is understandable and indeed shows the need for being tackled appropriately in a time when we have come to accept the biopsychosocial model of health care.

We therefore consider the variety of social, political and religious contexts that exist assess the claim that our understanding and teaching about end of life care is lacking. Whilst not entering the philosophical or legal debate about euthanasia, there is a force behind the euthanasia debate that reflects a failure of society to address this important issue.

This book (and its sister *Contemporary European Perspectives on the Ethics of End of Life Care*) was made possible (and supported with funding) by the Erasmus+ Project on End of life EndCare of the Bioethics Research Programme, Faculty of Medicine & Surgery, University of Malta. The partners were the Institute of Ethics, Dublin City University, and the Neurological Institute, Department of Biotechnological and Applied Clinical Sciences, University of L'Aquila. There were experts from law, philosophy, theology, bioethics, UNESCO and the Pontifical Academy for Life of the Vatican.

All authors are expert in their fields

Msida, Malta Pierre Mallia

Acknowledgements

This book is a direct result of the End-of-Life Erasmus+ Project *Harmonisation and Dissemination of Best Practice, Educating and alleviating concerns of Health Care Professionals on the proper practice of End Of Life. Project Reference: 2015-1-MT01-KA203-003728.* I would therefore like to thank the Project Support Office, especially Ms. Alexandra Attard and Ms Marilena Gauci of the University of Malta, and Mr. John Camilleri, Project Manager, who encouraged me to apply for the project and took care of all the red tape. I acknowledge the EUPA office, which manages Erasmus projects, and the partners of the project, Professor Francesca Pistoia of the Universita' dell-Aquila, Italy, and Professor Bert Gordijn of Dublin City University, Ireland, have been most helpful, as was our researcher Dr Nathan Emmerich.

Thanks are due also to the projects' guest participants: Prof. Henk ten Have, then at Duquesne University, Pittsburgh; Prof. Renzo Pegoraro, Chancellor of the Pontifical Academy for Life of the Vatican City; Prof. Anne-Marie Duguet, Paul Sabatier University, Toulouse; Dr Michael Bone, South Tyneside NHS Trust, UK; Dr Jurgen Abela and Dr Daniela Galea, University of Malta; Professor Alireza Bagheri, Tehran University and UNESCO International Bioethics Committee; Professor Chris Gastmans, Catholic University of Leuven; and finally Mr. Timothy Camilleri, administrating assistant.

An acknowledgement also goes to the editors of *Clinical Medicine* of the Royal College of Physicians, UK, for allowing us to reproduce images. It is impossible of course to mention all those who participated in the project, but a special thanks must go to the summer school participants in the partner countries who have contributed in many ways for developing ideas and sharing experiences. I would also like to thank the editors of the *Journal of the Malta College of Family Doctors* for the reproduction of the chapter by John Saunders on the Liverpool Care Pathway, presented as a prelude to the EndCare Erasmus+ project.

I would like to thank Prof. Henk ten Have, editor of the Springer Series on Global Ethics, who encouraged production of the book in this series. In this way, it reaches a global audience notwithstanding that end of life problems extend from well-developed to developing countries, albeit facing different problems as well. Last but not least, Mr. Christopher Wilby and Ms. Neelofar Yasmeen of Springer Nature who were invaluable in helping throughout the acceptance and production process.

Contents

About the Contributors

Gertrude Buttigieg is a licensed Speech Language Pathologist. Since 1995, Ms Buttigieg has practised in all areas of the profession from paediatric to geriatric care within a community and rehabilitation setting. Since June 2013 she has been recruited as Allied Health Practitioner (SLP) and Communications Officer with the Office of the Commissioner for Mental Health, Malta. On a voluntary basis she has been serving on the committee of the Association of Speech Language Pathologist since 1995. Between 2007 and 2018 she served as Honorary Secretary of the Malta Health Network and since April 2018 has been elected Chairperson of the Network. Since 2005 she has been serving as Honorary Secretary of the Malta Federation of Professional Associations. In 2014 she was elected on the Civil Society Committee of the Malta Council for Economic and Social Development as representative for the sectors of Health and Elderly. Ms Buttigieg is the elected member on the Malta Council for the Voluntary Sector for the sectors of health and disability. Gertrude has participated as speaker and participant in several conferences locally and abroad, lectured at local and foreign institutions. Over the past 10 years she has become a Patient advocate and has contribute to raise awareness on a national level of Patients' Rights and issues related to the Health sector such as patient education, patient empowerment, safety and access to services in an equitable and timely manner.

Sarah Cox, BSc, MBBS, FRCP, MSc, trained in medicine in London then specialised in Palliative Medicine being appointed to a new Consultant in Palliative Medicine post at Royal Trinity Hospice and Chelsea and Westminster Hospital in 1998. She is also an honorary Senior Lecturer at Imperial College London and an honorary consultant at Royal Hospital Chelsea (for the Chelsea Pensioners). Her clinical work is in the acute hospital setting and in the community. She has had a special interest in palliative care of non-malignant conditions, including HIV.

She is passionate about sharing good practice more widely and has designed an innovative simulation programme to develop the skills of generalists in recognising patients at the end of life and holding conversations about the future. She led on the expert reference group involved in developing and piloting a national data collection for palliative care including outcome measures. For the last **3** years she has lead a regional group to support improvements in palliative and end of life care across West London. Sarah chairs the Specialist Palliative Medicine group at the Royal College of Physicians and is an executive member of the national speciality group for Palliative Medicine in the UK and Ireland.

Dr Cox has taught in the end-of-life updates and courses of the Royal College of Physicians of London.

Nathan Emerich is a Postdoctoral Research Fellow in Ethics and End of Life Care at the Institute of Ethics, Dublin City University, and a Visiting Research Fellow at Queen's University Belfast. He has a background in Philosophy and took his PhD, which concerned the connection between the informal moral socialisation of medical students and their formal medical ethics education, under the supervision of medical sociologist. His work is interdisciplinary in nature and he has published on ethical expertise, social science research ethics and in bioethics more generally.

Anthony Fiorini, MB, ChB, FRCP, MD, M.Malt.St.(Melit), is the Clinical Chairperson of the Department of Geriatrics and a Consultant Geriatrician in the Department of Health, Malta. Being the first to hold such posts, he is considered instrumental in the setting up of hospital based geriatric services in Malta which include inter-professional team practices. He also holds the post of Visiting Senior Lecturer in the Department of Medicine and the Institute of Gerontology at the University of Malta and has been regularly involved in the teaching of both undergraduates and postgraduates of a number of disciplines, including the planning of courses, lecturing, giving tutorials and thesis tutoring. He has worked as a temporary consultant for the United Nations World Health Organisation visiting several countries to advise on the setting-up of services for the elderly and to participate in workshops and conferences. He has participated in, and coordinated courses, organised by the United Nations International Institute on Aging and has also acted as advisor to the Parliamentary Secretary for the Care of the Elderly in Malta. His is a co-founder and past chairperson of the Geriatric Medicine Society of Malta and has for a number of years sat on the full boards of both the European Union Geriatric Medicine Societies (EUGMS) and the European Union of Medical Specialists (UEMS – GMS). He is author of a number of peer-reviewed book chapters and journal articles and has regularly presented papers and chaired sessions at conferences both locally and abroad. He has acted as referee for both the *European Geriatric Journal* and the *Malta Medical Journal*. His main fields of interest include falls, services, team practice and medication management. His Doctorate thesis was based on the effectiveness of hospital-based assessment and rehabilitation geriatric units. His Masters dissertation was based on Maltese physicians who wrote poetry on doctoring.

Bert Grodijn, MA, PhD (Freiburg), PhD (Nijmegen), is Professor and Director of the Institute of Ethics at Dublin City University in Ireland. He has studied Philosophy and History in Utrecht, Strasbourg and Freiburg in Breisgau. In 1995 he was awarded a doctorate in Philosophy from the Albert-Ludwigs-Universität Freiburg, followed by a doctorate in Bioethics from the Radboud University Nijmegen in

2003. Bert has been a Visiting Professor at Lancaster University (UK), Georgetown University (USA), the National University of Singapore, the Fondation Brocher (Switzerland), and Yenepoya University (Mangalore, Karnataka, India). He has served on Advisory Panels and Expert Committees of the European Chemical Industry Council, the European Patent Organisation, the Irish Department of Health and UNESCO. Bert is Editor-in-Chief of two book series: The International Library of Ethics, Law and Technology and Advances in Global Bioethics as well as a peer-reviewed journal: *Medicine, Health Care and Philosophy*, all published by Springer Nature. He is Secretary of the European Society for Philosophy of Medicine and Healthcare and President of the International Association of Education in Ethics.

Pierre Mallia, MD, MPhil, MA (Law), FRCP, FRCGP, PhD, is Professor of Family Medicine and Patients' Rights in the Faculty of Medicine & Surgery at the Medical School, Mater Dei Hospital, where he also coordinates the Bioethics Research Programme. He is Consultant in Clinical Ethics at Malta's main hospital 'Materi Dei'. He is Chairperson and founder of the Medicine & Law Programme of the Faculty of Laws within the same university and a Visiting Professor at the Laennec University of Lyon, France. He is Chairman of the Health Ethics Committee of the Department of Health and recently has been made Chairperson of the National Bioethics Consultative Committee of the Ministry of Health, where he has been advisor to the several consecutive Ministers. He has recently been also appointed Chairman of the Faculty Research Ethics Committee (FREC) of the Faculty of Medicine & Surgery at the University of Malta.

At the moment he is the Principal Investigator and holder of the Erasmus + EndCare project, which is studying issues and problems of applying pathways at the end of life. He represents the University of Malta as the Principal partner, along with two other partner countries (Italy and Ireland) and experts from the UK, Ireland, France, Iran, Toronto, USA, and the Pontifical Academy for Life of the Vatican. He is planning a second project which will involve Patient Groups and Palliative Care organisations.

He has published over 80 articles in international peer-reviewed journals and also several books including one by Springer Nature, The Nature of the Doctor Patient Relationship. He has contributed Chapters to Springer's Encylopedia of Global Ethics (3 Vols), and to Springer's Handbook for global ethics (4 Vols), edited by Professors Henk Ten Have and Bert Gordijn.

Piret Paal, PhD, MA, BA (b. 1977 in Estonia), is a Reader in Nursing Science (Palliative Care) and Deputy Director of the WHO Collaborating Centre at the Institute of Nursing Science and Practice, Paracelsus Medical University, Salzburg, Austria. Since 2017, she has provided technical support to the World Health Organization (WHO) Regional Office for Europe (WHO EURO) to strengthen palliative care at member states in Europe. She is involved in palliative care education related projects, such as EDUPALL (undergraduate medical education), NurseEduPal (undergraduate nursing education), Pd_Pal (neuropalliative care).

She teaches global health, palliative care and spiritual care. She is a steering group member of European Association for Palliative Care (EAPC) Educational Reference Group and the INPCS Education Committee at the International Neuropalliative Care Society (INPCS).

Paul Paes, MBBS, MSc, MMEd, EdD, FRCP, SFHEA, is a Consultant in Palliative Medicine, based in Northumbria Healthcare Foundation Trust. Alongside his clinical role, he led the integration of palliative care services in the trust until 2015, including the creation of innovative hospital inpatient Palliative Care Units, the Marie Curie @ Northumbria joint venture and a 7-day rapid response service. End of Life services in the trust were rated as 'Outstanding' by the Care Quality Commission in 2016.

His leadership roles include being Clinical Director of the Northumberland New Models of Care Vanguard Programme as part of the NHS Five Year Forward View, and now Clinical Director of community services. He is currently working with colleagues in the NHS and voluntary sectors and Universities to set up a research and transformation programme to complement and drive improvement in clinical services.

He is also active in research and education, holding a joint post with Newcastle University. His research interests are around decision making- he has recently completed his own doctorate on practical wisdom, and his doctoral students have carried out studies in decision making in palliative care. He has contributed e-learning sessions and book chapters in Advance Care Planning and Palliative Care.

His other main interest is in medical education; he is Sub-Dean in the School of Medical Education, Newcastle University, with responsibility for Admissions. He sits on the Executive Committee of the Association for Palliative Medicine and chairs the Education Committee. He has taught in the end-of-life updates and courses of the Royal College of Physicians of London.

Renzo Pegoraro is a medical doctor and a moral theologian He is Professor of Bioethics at Theological Faculty of North-East of Italy, University of Pavoda. He is President of the Research Ethics Committee of the Venetian Oncological Institute and has been Scientific Director of Fondazione Lanza in Padova for 20 years. The Foundation does research into Bioethical Issues and has hosted conferences and produced numerous publications. He is also past President of European Society of Philosophy of Medicine and Healthcare (ESPMH) and past President of European Association of Centers of Medical Ethics (EACME). In 2011 he was appointed Chancellor of the Pontifical Academy for Life in Rome and travels between Rome and Pavoda.

Francesca Pistoia, MD, PhD, completed her degree summa cum laude in medicine and surgery, and thereafter specialised in neurology summa cum laude, at the University of L'Aquila. She earned a PhD in Internal Medicine and Applied Immunology at the same University. Currently she holds the position of Assistant Professor of Neurorehabilitation at the University of L'Aquila. So far, she has contributed to 95 papers (83 in peer-reviewed international journals and 12 on Italian journals); 80 papers are indexed in Pubmed). She also presented her results at national and international congresses (resulting in 71 abstracts and communications). H-index (Scopus): 21. Her research is mainly focused on the topic of *diagnosis, prognosis and rehabilitation of patients with severe brain injury* with the aim of implementing validated assessment tools to identify physical, cognitive and behavioural disabilities and quantify rehabilitation-related outcomes. Research topics include: the evaluation of patients with disorders of consciousness (vegetative state and minimally conscious state) as a consequence of severe brain injury: her studies in this area have been aimed at evaluating the neurobiological and behavioural factors, which may influence the recovery of consciousness, and the implementation of new therapeutical approaches including brain computer interfaces; the identification of disorders of motor imagery and the perception of emotions in patients with locked-in syndrome. She also contributed to research addressing the epidemiology of cerebrovascular diseases and of Parkinson's disease in population-based registries, and the role of comorbidities in headache pathogenesis and of behavioural therapies in patients with chronic headache. She serves as a member of the Ethical Committee of the University of L'Aquila.

John Saunders, MA (Wales), MA (UCL), MD (Lond), FRCP, is Consultant Physician at Nevill Hall Hospital, Abergavenny, South Wales. He was the former Chairman of the Committee for Ethical Issues in Medicine of the Royal College of Physicians of London and is an Honorary Professor in Philosophy, History and Law in Healthcare at the School of Health Science, Swansea University, Wales, UK. Professor Saunders is a highly respected physician and ethicist and has contributed to the development of ethics in the UK in several ways including invitations to write articles, as Chair of the RCP Ethics Committee and is referred to frequently in many publications and journals, including the British Medical Journal. In the beginning of the EndCare (Erasmus +) project, he was invited to Malta by the coordinator and chief editor of this volume to give a talk on the lessons learnt from the failure of the Liverpool Care Pathway in the UK. He was an advisor during the EndCare Project. He has edited the 2019 edition of *Ethics and Communication, in the Medicine (Elsevier)*, a CME series for specialisation in Medicine.

Andrew Thorns, MBBS, MA, MRCGP, FRCP, has been a consultant in palliative medicine holding a joint post between Pilgrims Hospices and the East Kent Hospitals University Foundation Trust, based mainly at Queen Elizabeth the Queen Mother Hospital in Margate since 2000.

He has been Director of Medicine for Pilgrims Hospice since August 2015.

For over 10 years he ran an MSc programme at the University of Kent, leading on the research and ethics modules.

He remains a member of the research group hosted by the Centre for Health Service Studies which strives to increase research in the locality.

Andrew has a keen interest in ethical issues at the end of life following on from the master's programme, in particular the use of sedation and opioids and the place of cardiopulmonary resuscitation. He is a facilitator for the Connected advanced communication skills course. He is widely published in the field of palliative care in international peer-reviewed journals and is a regular speak of end-of-life courses and seminars at the Royal College of Physicians of London.

Christopher Vella, is a healthcare professional and bioethicist within the private sector who has been involved with medical ethics, policy and management. For the past years he has been involved in setting up and running his own private laboratory, whilst also pursuing his passion for medical ethics and law by providing consultation services and policy compliancy audits and reviews in the private sector. After obtaining his MA in Medical ethics and Law he got involved in the Maltese Voluntary sector, with the aim to promote patient rights and contribute to patient advocacy. He is currently serving as secretary in the Malta Health Network (MHN), where he represents them on the Universal Access to Healthcare core group of the EPF amongst other things. As of 2018 he is currently undergoing post-graduate studies in Genetic and Genomic Counselling.

Dominique Wakefield is a Consultant in Palliative Medicine working at Guy's and St Thomas' NHS Foundation Trust in London. She has worked in a number of developing countries and has an interest in healthcare delivery in low resource settings. Dr Wakefield holds an Honorary Senior Lecturer post with the Cicely Saunders Institute of Palliative Care, Policy and Rehabilitation, King's College London. Having undertaken her clinical academic training at the Cicely Saunders Institute she went onto develop an interest in leadership, completing a Clinical Management Fellowship and Executive Master's in Medical Leadership with Cass Business School, University of London. She is the honorary secretary for the Royal Society of Medicine's Palliative Care Section, supporting the delivery of postgraduate education and learning.

Part I
Ethical and Social Issues

Chapter 1
Introduction: Harmonising End of Life Care – A Global Public Health Issue

Pierre Mallia, Nathan Emmerich, Bert Gordijn, and Francesca Pistoia

Abstract End of life care is a global problem. From Western societies where death has been medicalised to lack of availability of palliative care which has led to an increase in the demand for euthanasia, to developing countries where end of life is affected by lack of resources including hospitals, home care, water problems and poverty. End of Life (EoL) care is a field in which, notwithstanding moral agreement on most issues, continues globally to be a source of controversy and uncertainty. This chapter looks at end of life as a global public health issues as described by the World Health Organisation. As an introduction to the texts, it puts end of life in perspective of global concerns and reviews the chapters in the book which have the aim of together attempting to provide a model for end of life care which can effectively be implemented globally, giving perspectives from learned experiences, systems, cultures, professional issues, medico-legal proposals, and pathways to implement change. A summary of these is given as an introduction to the reader.

Keywords End of life · Global · Ethical and social issues · Medico-legal proposals · Pathways

P. Mallia (✉)
Medical School, University of Malta, Msida, Malta
e-mail: pierre.mallia@um.edu.mt

N. Emmerich
Australian National University, Canberra, Australia

B. Gordijn
Institute of Ethics, Dublin City University, Dublin, Ireland

F. Pistoia
Neurological Institute, University of L'Aquila, Coppito, L'Aquila, Italy

P. Mallia et al. (eds.), *Challenges to the Global Issue of End of Life Care*, Advancing Global Bioethics 17, https://doi.org/10.1007/978-3-030-86386-9_1

The World Health Organisation has recognised end of life as a public health and a global issue. There is growing concern about the provision of palliative care between developed and developing countries. A 'common global future' for palliative care across the globe on the other hand, must take into consideration the divergent cultural issues and what is meant by a 'good death'. This is not to overlook the fact that there are also wide variations between individuals and between communities. In many western countries, for example, there are cultural groups who view death in different ways, underpinning differences in goals.

Many people die in developing countries without adequate pain relief. Moreover, especially in developed countries, improvement in chronic disease treatment and cancer care has prolonged life. However, death by no means is a harmonious process in these countries, with many asserting the medicalization of death and indeed its undue prolongation. This is mostly due to false hopes and lack of awareness of moral issues both within hospitals and the public. Social institutions must enter the debate in a positive way rather than merely opposing technology and euthanasia. Because of this clouding of what we want death to be like, many are in danger, or have, been pushed into vegetative states at most, or at the very least a prolonged dying process.

There are many issues which define the quality of end of life care on a global level ranging from poverty and lack of basic resources to lack of a proper functioning structure to provide a 'good death'. We mean to define 'harmonisation' as how one can address issues within institutions or in countries which are not allowing good end of life care to be implemented. End of life care has become a problem in many countries. In some it has been medicalised. In other there are even basic resources at hand. Health professionals have not only a moral duty to their patients but are strategically placed to improve, even by providing evidence, care within their institution or country. For this we need good models to bring professionals together and to engage them with the relevant authorities and people. This expands their work meaningfully as patient advocates and facilitators for proper change.

Conversely there is a growing concern of medical neglect of dying people globally. This ranges from the growing concern of increase in futile treatment and the death-denying culture of developed countries, to lack of pain relief and basic palliative care in developing countries. In fact, 85% of annual deaths occur in developing countries. Moreover, the population of the world is increasing with the process of death becoming more extended as life-threatening diseases are transformed into chronic diseases and terminal illnesses lasting several years. It is this which turns end of life into a public health factor and therefore a global issue.

Global disparity means that problems within institutions vary. Moreover, within the same country, even developed ones, health professions in one hospital may have or assert different needs than others. These may range from communication issues with patients, implementation of cultural divergences awareness, lack of human resources, and lack of inter-professional communication or agreement. These require a strategy to tackle. The book aims to help professionals tackle both institutional issues and also issues which are related to the whole country they work in, bring them together to work towards improving health systems, which, at the end of the day, end of life care depends upon.

The number of popular books published by experienced health care professionals showing their frustrations in the field is testament to the medicalisation of end of life care in hospital (Gawande 2015; Warraich 2017). This has mostly to do with the developed world but it is not only a lesson for developing countries but actually provides hope to more impoverished ones that resources need not be as hefty as one might at first think when considering end of life as a public health issue. The increase in the amount of literature on end of life by doctors and other health professionals involved at the end of life and dealing with the discontent the profession feels about the incoherent way we treat dying people shows that this has affected the existential nature of health care professionals. Anything which makes us question whether we are doing something right or wrong, or not sufficiently well can be called to affect the meaning of one's work: Ought we to keep them alive as much as possible? When ought we to stop nutrition and even hydration? When is it a discomfort? Many have the conviction that we should at least provide hydration. And indeed, most people dying in hospital do so with a drip attached to them. Yet when someone dies at home it is accepted that this is not always possible. Is hydration a part of dying naturally? Does it really provide the comfort we think it does? Are we convinced that a doctor on call who is asked to change a drip on a dying patient ought to puncture the patient a number of times trying to find a vein which is not collapsed? Are we convinced that these patients do not feel that pain? Who makes the call to stop hydration nowadays? Even when we stop nutrition, doctors and nurses may disagree with other health care professionals who may insist on nutrition via a PEG. These people will eventually need to evacuate their bowel. But, do dying people need nutrition in their last days? Most people who die naturally do so without food. It is appropriate in conscious or semiconscious patients, but doubtful otherwise. But it is a fact that we may not be preparing patients and relatives and indeed ourselves that dying people do not need nutrition and that this may simply be prolonging the agony. As the GMC guidelines recommend, we need to recognise the imminence of death and move towards a plan so as not to come towards the end with doubts on whether to increase morphine due to the fear of respiratory suppression to even whether re-inserting an intravenous line or a subcutaneous drip to provide fluids is necessary when we are expecting the patient to die very soon.

Tackling these problems is the subject of this book whilst providing a model for harmonising end of life care within the context of one's institution or country. It follows a European Union Erasmus + project on End of Life (Erasmus+, ENDCARE) (Mallia 2015–2018) which had the aim of educating health professionals and social institutions on how to manage these issues.[1] Many hospitals, for example, face

[1]The End Care Erasmus+ Project started with the realisation that end of life care is not homogenous notwithstanding that we have ample moral sources to harmonise it. End of life care has become medicalised. Many have come to expect nothing less than miraculous cures even when people suddenly approach an unexpected death. A consultant recently told me that when faced with a patient who was dying a discussion arose with one of his registrars who had come from the UK and who had suggested the Liverpool Care Pathway, which was intended to be nothing more than a Palliative Care pathway for the dying and accepted in the NICE guidelines. The consultant replied that in Malta Euthanasia is not accepted. One cannot blame him as the LCP turned out not

problems with communication, with advance care planning, and dealing with unrealistic expectations. Many health professionals of course do not come from a philosophical background and would not understand, for example, the moral equivalence principle between omitting to start treatment and withdrawing treatment which is being given, the latter being seen more emotionally charged. This shows that end of life is not merely a philosophical problem but goes in the realm of the psychosocial. Globally different needs are asserted and the text hopes to serve as a resource for health care professionals to tackle issues without feeling helpless. There is a sea between theoretical bioethics, which gives us the necessary grounding of our moral actions, and clinical ethics when one is faced with a real patient and real relative; and not least a team which not only wants to do well by the patient but want to be seen to be doing what is just.

The book has four sections. The first tackles ethical and social issues. John Saunders (Chap. 2) takes a look at the Liverpool Care Pathway and discusses how a good model turned into a poorly implemented one. We stress it is important to learn such lessons before trying to improve end of life care. Indeed, this was a clear case where the road to hell was paved by very good intentions. This chapter identifies the strengths and weaknesses one can find in the provision of proper EoL care. Some instructions may be strong in one area and weak in another and it is important to identify these in order to harmonise end of life for patients. In some areas of a country one may have hospices, whilst in poorer areas one does not. This has been the experience with the Liverpool Care Pathway, which was meant to be a palliative care pathway similar to the one provided in hospices but which could have been provided in hospitals. Yet its weaknesses were in retrospect seen to be lack of proper training. The pathway on its own was not enough. The author discusses how strengths and weaknesses ought to be identified before they become problematic. The author traces the problems of the Liverpool Care Pathway showing good intentions can be misinterpreted and misused.

Renzo Pegoraro (Chap. 3) discusses how religious and social teaching affects both the understanding of patients and of their relatives. Institutions such as religions and can play an active role in promoting what is allowed at the end of life and

to be applied with proper training and became a tick-box where all people who were put on the pathways suddenly had all treatment, hydration and nutrition stopped. This of course was a misapplication, as all know, of the pathway and led to the 'One chance to get it right' document. It was a learning experience. People were simply abandoned on a 'pathway' which was meant to provide them with proper end of life care as was done in Hospices throughout the UK. The pathway was developed for those people who did not have access to hospices. It turned out not to have been practiced as a pathway.

Preliminary studies carried out did show that many doctors are concerned about legal issues and lack of understanding of relatives of what ought to be done. It is with this understanding that this project involved not only the Faculty of Medicine & Surgery of the University of Malta but also the Faculties of Laws and of Theology; the former to give us the legal guidance, the lack of which was complained about and the latter to remind us of the accepted moral practice. The EndCare (Erasmus+) project also partnered with Dublin City University and the University of L'Aquila, besides experts from law, philosophy, theology, bioethics and institutions like UNESCO and the Pontifical Academy for Life of the Vatican.

educating people that this is charitable towards someone who is dying. Death is not the intended outcome here; it is simply the inevitable outcome and one want to make the process the least burdensome as possible. Spiritual care at the EoL is always seen of utmost importance. This may range from religious customs to the existential questions which people facing death are confronted with. Spirituality goes beyond religion. Yet there are also important consistencies between various denominations and religions which ought to be understood, especially in societies which are becoming more multicultural in order to address the needs of the populations. It is hoped that this chapter emphasises upon readers the importance of the educational role of religious institutions and the implications of its lack thereof.

In Chap. 4, Paal Piret discusses global systems in palliative care. This chapter gives an insight into various difficulties, problems and the state of the art of palliative care around the globe. The chapter draws, amongst others, on the World Palliative Care Alliance (WPCA) which is a global action network focussing on hospice and palliative care development worldwide and has done work to identify what the problems are contextually. The chapter reviews the need of palliative care worldwide, existing models of palliative care, available resources, including financial, philanthropic, research support and education, the main barriers to palliative care, and the necessary responses. Importantly, the chapter discusses how the contents of the book fit in these situations. In Chap. 5, Pierre Mallia discusses what is usually meant by 'a good death'. There is considerable talk in the literature about this. It has been the topic of a day course held in 2016 at the Royal College of Physicians in London. Doctors, health professionals and patients may not be aware that people have different views about what a good death is. The place where one dies is not necessarily of great importance as people attach. The author discusses some studies in this regard and explains what many would consider a 'good death'. One cannot improve end of life car without considering this important psychosocial issue.

In section two we tackle professional issues keeping in the global context of topics. Andrew Thorn and Dominique Wakefield (Chap. 6) discuss Medical decision-making at the end of life within the global context. It is recognised that many doctors may be specialised in different areas but this does not mean that they necessarily have the necessary training in palliative care. Whilst there are many places that have palliative care hospitals and hospitals having palliative care units, the process of recognition of imminence of death starts from as early as a year before. In this situation palliative care may not have yet started. The training of doctors in managing patients who are going to die, especially where there is no palliative care unit, and in making decisions at the end of life is discussed.

Conversely General Practitioners / family doctors face end of life on a regular basis. Pierre Mallia (Chap. 7) discusses how family medicine changes according to country but how the GP can contribute to end of life when people wish to die at home. Whilst some people have arrangements to die at home and therefore require regular visits by the family doctor, others need the services of GPs to help from the very beginning when a diagnosis of a terminal illness is made. The chapter discusses the work of general practitioners and how they can help families and patients with services and indeed start the process of planning ahead. Post graduate curricula on the topic of end of life are discussed, especially for the case of the UK, and what is expected from a general practitioner.

Inter-professional issues are a fact of life. Anthony Fiorini discusses in Chap. 8 how team approaches can be made to work from his experience in being a consultant and director of a hospital for elderly people. Doctors and nurses work together but they come from different backgrounds of training and their work, whilst complimentary is very different. Nurses can be found on a ward for the whole of their duty hours, whilst doctors may be seen only in ward rounds and when they visit patients. The team approach may not be easy. A model of a team approach, which has been very successful, is discussed within the context of a hospital for elderly that deals with EoL amongst others. The value of having multidisciplinary meetings after ward rounds has proved to be very successful and the process is discussed.

In Chap. 9, Sarah Cox deals with managing difficult conversations through a culturally sensitive approach. Conflict inevitably arises towards the end of life. This is understandable as families face the death of a loved one. However, there may be disagreement on what health care professionals think is actually beneficial for the patient and what the wishes of the family or patient are. The chapter gives communication issues with patients and how conflict can be managed. This illustrates the importance of training for health professionals in this regard even when there are proper pathways in place, recognising the distress that people go through.

The third section deals with the important issues touching upon the medico-legal framework. Many health professionals fear that any decision they make, even if morally acceptable can be seen by the relatives as shortening intentionally the life of their loved one and the fear of litigation may therefore lead to sub-optimal care. Many witness patients dying in pain and this should not be the case in these days. Cultures, religious institutions, patient groups, and others can be instrumental in imparting proper advice to the population in order for them to understand their rights and indeed what is meant by futility, disproportionate treatment, right to refuse life prolonging treatment, etc. There are many misconceptions among the general population, such as that pain relief which can hasten death is a form of euthanasia and therefore extrapolate from this a ‘why not in other situations’ attitude. Social teaching may provide in simple language what cultures and religious denomination accept and why.

Paul Paes (Chap. 10) discusses the important issue of Advanced Care Planning (ACP) on a global level. This chapter is dealt with in this section due to its contrast to Advance Directive, which are usually legal documents and in turn need a legislative framework for recognition. Conversely ACPs are discussions with patients and notes are made in the file. Whilst laws have to be respected, one has documented what the patient wishes. Paes discusses issues with refusal of treatment and describes the difference between futile treatment and treatment which may not be futile but is considered disproportionate and/or extraordinary. Moreover, there may be the misconception that it is not the patient who decides for himself or herself what is considered extraordinary. In order to commence advanced planning one needs to recognise the imminence of death and plan ahead with the patient. This involves appropriate communication, which need formal training, just as doctors and nurses learn how to take a history. It also requires formally recoding wishes and good communication. Having the appropriate opening statements and questions serves as a tool to engage appropriately with patients and relatives. However, one recognises that conflict may often arise with relatives and in these days, unless we are to return to paternalistic models and also face many legal issues, health professionals must be able to understand the nature of conflict and know how to resolve it. We note that Advanced Care Planning already happens to a certain extend by GPs when people decide to die at home. Family doctors know when to stop treatment because they explain its futility in the presence of relatives and at a time convenient to them. They speak with relatives and explain when 'time has come'. But they are at an advantage. The GP has known the family for quite some time; there is a fiduciary relationship built over years. It is not the same in a hospital where personnel work in shifts and where decision are made perhaps only during ward rounds, ideas can vary on whether we should keep that drip, even at least subcutaneously, whilst someone has to make a decision alone whilst on duty.

The proper training of physician in palliative care is becoming more and more important. This is discussed in Chap. 11 by Francesca Pistoia. The need for this is felt both in the primary care and secondary care setting. EoL care cannot be taken for granted and knowledge of the morality and basic medical attention is not enough. It can be shown, for example, that the care is not harmonised with one physician insisting on a continuous form of hydration whilst another recognises that this may become burdensome. From a medical point of view standards of care need to be followed which, from the biological aspect, and not perhaps from the psycho-social one, must be in harmony so as to provide all patients with individuals trained in palliative care, even though they may be specialist in another major area. Universal palliative care training at both undergraduate and graduate levels of education will surely decrease any litigation as consistency of practice (harmonisation) will be reached.

Finally, Nathan Emmerich (Chap. 12) discusses whether palliative sedation poses a real dilemma. Palliative sedation has been at the centre of debate recently and even seen as a path tantamount to euthanasia. Although one may use any form of treatment not following a standard of care (and therefore negligently and even criminally), when following clear guidelines there ought not to be any ethical dilemma. The hype around palliative sedation may be therefore misplaced and its place in proper palliative care should find itself comfortably. There ought to be a combination of pain relief and sedation in some instances, and indeed a patient may evidence a choice if pain relief does not provide the necessary comfort. Also, there are levels of sedation which are addressed. We note that the Liverpool Care Pathway had good guidance on this but lack of appropriate training led to its misguided use tying this chapter with the previous one.

The final section deals with a model for implementing and harmonising end of life care within an institution. It discusses in its various chapters how to implement and organise seminar or retreats where professionals can express their concerns in a protected environment and together form a plan to understand the underlying issues, whether there are protocols, and whether any administrative changes need to be implemented. Different settings will have different needs. Some may find they need appropriate protocols; some may find they need to tackle administrative issues; other more legal and social issues, such as educating the public. How to engage with these is important and, in this regard, we discuss therefore the curriculum for such meetings and how pathways are implemented and followed up.

Health professionals have a moral duty to improve care. Often however they may feel this is beyond their control. But it can be done by working together with patients' groups, social institutions, politicians, and legislators. It is not a quick-fix task. Indeed, it may be slow. But we are sure it will provide broader meaning to health professionals dealing with the broader issues in order to help them with the individual patient. We believe that this text will go beyond an academic perspective therefore and helps professionals: 1. to reinforce quality end of life care as a global public health issue, 2. to strengthen the capacity to improve end of life care utilizing resources available, whilst 3. to develop pathways towards improved strategies. ALL chapters view end of life through the global lens.

Engaging patient groups in implementing improvement to end of life care is a topic discussed by Gertrude Buttigieg and Christopher Vella (Chap. 13). The authors how patients can be involved in various aspects of health care, including end of life management. Patients are the appropriate group to ask what matters at the end of life. They can help considerable in improving not only management and palliative care, but even what drugs they would wish to be developed.

Finally, Pierre Mallia (Chap. 14) discusses how to develop pathways to improve EoL care and Advanced Planning Globally, bring health care professionals together to identify problems and formulate pathways a curriculum for training. A curriculum is a live animal and changes according to needs. It is not merely a syllabus; neither is it meant to simply train people in specific areas such as morality or palliative care. Rather the curriculum discussed is a tool for institutions to get stakeholders together to discuss what are the strengths, weaknesses, opportunities and threats of EoL care where it is deemed not to be working effectively. It discusses how issues such as lack of moral education, lack of an infrastructure for proper communication, and lack of legislative frameworks which can help health care professionals, and other areas, can be tackled and strategies developed to tackle the in situ needs of the institution (or country) in which the problem is identified. The curriculum can be used in places such as summer schools or retreats and looks at inter- and intra-professional issues, hospital management, social and political issues, and indeed primary care and the role it can play. A model of how this is working in a Mediterranean country is discussed and how the model is adaptable on a global perspective. The curriculum is the ore one which has to be implemented by people working within a context and who understand the local scenario in order to work towards addressing not only the issues but the public concerned, be they politicians, administrators, patients, and special institutions such as religious teachers and churches.

EoL continues to provide its fair share of problems and dilemmas. Training is something which is necessary in continuing professional development plans and public teaching of the ethical issues at EoL have to continuously be complimentary. The Erasmus End of Life (EndCare) project has identified this concern and created a curriculum as a tool to help institutions. The chapter summarises the salient features of the book and the conclusion the various authors have reached and discusses the strengths, opportunities and any threats of using a model which can address a global end of life care.

References

Gawande, A. 2015. *Being mortal. Illness, medicine, and what matters in the end.* London: Profile Books in association with Wellcome Collection.

Mallia, P. 2015–2018, *EndCare. On Harmonisation and dissemination of good practice at the end-of-life.* Project no. 2015-1-MT01-KA203-003728.

Warraich, H. 2017. *Modern death. How medicine changed the end of life.* London: Duckworth Overlook.

Chapter 2
The Liverpool Care Pathway: Lessons in Care of the Dying

John Saunders

Abstract The importance of this chapter is to learn from the experience of the Liverpool Care Pathway in the UK. The lessons are evident from inception to perception and ought to be a lesson globally, especially in countries where the population does not know enough about the values, especially with regard to their cultural and/or religious beliefs, about what is morally permitted and what is in fact euthanasia. The LCP provided grounds for concern because of lack of communication with patients and relatives and also because of lack of training in palliative care and thus perhaps affecting the application of the pathway. The name itself, both as 'pathway' and the Liverpool Care Pathway', is indeed awkward as it seems a 'pathway' to death. It was thus attacked that it was a pathway to end the lives of patients. Notwithstanding this the pathways itself was strongly recommended by the NICE guidelines and indeed supported by most Colleges of physicians and other specialities. It is a lesson which ought to be recognised globally so as not to waste resources and energy only to find a good protocol being attacked.

Education of the public through state, doctors, and other institutions (including religions and Churches), involvement of society, key explanation to relatives and indeed education of health care professionals in the use of the pathway is the key message from the LVP. After the Saga, Professor John Saunders, then chairman of the Royal College of Physicians of London was invited to Malta to discuss what went wrong with the palliative care pathway which, as noted, was accepted in the NICE guidelines. The pathways came under attack, most notably from a Maltese physician working in the UK as being a 'euthanasia' pathway. This was the main reason Professor Saunders was invited to Malta. Of course, euthanasia was not the case but the misapplication of the pathways, by simply using it as a tick box and immediately without due deliberation removing, for example, any treatment, did make the pathway a danger when used by those not appropriately trained in Palliative

---

J. Saunders (✉)
College of Health and Human Sciences, Swansea University, Swansea, UK

Committee for Ethical Issues in Medicine, Royal College of Physicians of London & Consultant Physician, Nevill Hall Hospital, Abergavenny, UK
e-mail: saundersjohn@doctors.org.uk

P. Mallia et al. (eds.), *Challenges to the Global Issue of End of Life Care*, Advancing Global Bioethics 17, https://doi.org/10.1007/978-3-030-86386-9_2

care. This article was one by invitation by the Journal of the Malta College of Family Doctors. It also appeared in the proceedings on the conference organised by one of the editors of this book.

Professor Saunders explains the necessity and the soundness of the pathway whilst showing that the bad implementation of even a good thing can have bad consequences if not supervised well. The history of this pathway should be well understood by those intending to implement change. The article looks at the pitfalls offers sound advice. The article, reproduced with a few changes by the author and with the permission of the above-mentioned journal is an important lesson, especially coming from the United Kingdom, which has had considerable influence in the introduction of Palliative care through the efforts of Dame Cicely Saunders, and indeed the global influence that British medicine has.

Keywords End of life · Liverpool care pathway · 'Pathway of death' · Neuberger inquiry · National debate

2.1 At the End of Life

For many practising doctors, especially in general practice or in general internal medicine, decisions at the end of life are often some of the most difficult. Not only is decision making difficult, but implementation may create a further set of problems. Most of us are orientated to *doing* something – usually something that is active, promoting life or health. Many end of life decisions demand something different: the acceptance that life is coming to an end and that the quality of the final phase of the patient's illness is to offer a good death. The doctor must re-orientate his or her thinking to a different, less distinct target. Yet the old aphorism still rings true that the aim of medicine is to cure sometimes, to alleviate often and to comfort always, (guérir quelquefois, soulager souvent, consoler toujours).[1]

As an aside, the origin of this saying is uncertain; it is associated with Dr. EL Trudeau and inscribed on his statue in the grounds of the Trudeau Institute at Saranac Lake New York and also on the fireplace beneath an oil painting in the library. But it is found too in a window in the New York Academy of Medicine and variously attributed to Oliver Wendell Holmes, Paré, Florence Nightingale and Hippocrates.

Within that aphorism, comes the need to understand 'comfort' in terms of ultimate aims and desires: the explanation or meaning attached to the illness experience. Comfort is different from alleviation in this respect. A book such as Jeremy Taylor's '*The Rule and Exercises of Holy living, holy dying*' of 1651 sets out what is comforting in mortal illness. From Taylor's perspective, this is unashamedly religious: reflections on the brevity of life, length of years, charity and alms, fear of

[1] Payne LM. "Guérir quelquefois, Soulager souvent, Consoler toujours" BMJ; 1967;**4**:47–8.

death, hope of heaven. Comfort is here not symptom relief, but a more positive view of life's ending. Similarly in Tolstoy's novella '*Ivan Illich*', the comfort is the light: 'In place of death there was light' 'So that's what it is! What joy!' And Illich escapes from his 'black hole'.

For a previous generation, the increased place of technology in medicine often seemed to have displaced the willingness to sit by the bedside and wait. Senior doctors in particular often rushed by, ignoring the needs of those who had moved beyond the stage of curative or even alleviative medicine. It was forgotten that 'they also serve who only stand and wait.[2]' The dying patient was moved into a side-ward where he or she would not be seen, sometimes ignored by all but the most junior doctor on the team. Outside hospital, it was the nurses in the community who played the key role in care. Medicine had forgotten something of its vocation. It was into the world of this (admittedly sweeping) generalisation, that the new specialty of palliative medicine was born – its chief midwife that remarkable nurse, social worker and doctor, Cicely Saunders.[3] From a UK perspective, the hospice movement – spearheaded in the east end of London in St Joseph's Hospice and in south London in St Christopher's – rapidly gained momentum. It received strong support from the voluntary sector, especially Christian organisations, but as it grew also gained grant support from government. The work of Saunders in her concept of 'total pain' was important, as was the adoption of the WHO's subsequent definition[4] of palliative care as 'total active care':

> Palliative care is the active total care of patients whose disease is not responsive to curative treatment. Control of pain, of other symptoms and of psychological, social and spiritual problems is paramount. The goal of palliative care is achievement of the best possible quality of life for patients and their families.

The benefits of hospice care, with support from dedicated professionals, became obvious enough. Yet it was clear that hospice provision could not be extended to all dying patients. In the UK, those dying in hospices make up less than 5% of total deaths. The lessons of the hospice had to extend beyond its walls to other institutions – principally hospitals, but also to those dying at home or in residential care homes or nursing homes. This led to the development of the Liverpool Care Pathway for the dying patient (LCP).

The LCP was the product of a collaboration in 2004 between the University of Liverpool, Marie Curie Cancer Care and the Royal Liverpool and Broadgreen University Hospitals NHS Trust – that is to say, a collaboration between the voluntary sector, academia and the UK's National Health Service. The pathway continued to be a focus of collaborative work with various national organisations, including the National Council for Palliative Care, the Royal College of Physicians and the

[2] Milton J. On his blindness. Poems 1655.

[3] Saunders C. A personal therapeutic journey. BMJ 1996;313: 1599.

[4] World Health Organisation Expert Committee. Cancer pain relief and palliative care. Geneva: WHO, 1990:11.

Care Quality Commission.[5] The LCP had both a national and international programme and had a role in the provision of end of life care in at least 17 countries. Its primary aim was to improve care in the last hours or days of life – that is to say, it was not a programme for terminal illness overall, but for its final stages. Cicely Saunders herself said:

> All the careful details of the pathway are a salute to the enduring worth of an individual life. Such an ending can help those left behind to pick up the threads of memory and begin to move forward.[6]

As the Marie Curie Institute states, the LCP was recognized as a model of best practice in the NHS Beacon Programme (2001), incorporated into the National End of Life Care Programme (2004–7), recommended in the National Institute of Clinical Excellence guidance in 2004[7] and recommended in the End of Life Care Strategy by the English Department of Health in 2008. For the dying patient, it was thought by those with expertise in palliative medicine to represent the best standard of care.

2.2 The Pathway[8]

A pathway is a complex intervention for the mutual decision making and organization of care processes for a well-defined group of patients during a well-defined period – in this case, those with a prognosis of days or hours of life only. Its five key elements consisted of.

- An explicit statement of goals or of the key elements of care based on evidence & best practice
- The facilitation of the communication among team members and with patients and families.
- The coordination of the care process by coordinating the roles and sequencing the activities o the multi-disciplinary team (MDT), patients and carers.
- The documentation, monitoring and evaluation of variances and outcomes
- The identification of the appropriate resources.

The advice in the Liverpool Care Pathway document was entirely compatible with other end of life guidance, which it supplements. In the UK, this includes

[5] http://www.liv.ac.uk/mcpcil/about-us/

[6] Saunders C. In: Ellershaw J, Wilkinson S. Care of the dying: a pathway to excellence. 2nd ed 2011, Oxford University Press, Oxford.

[7] See: End of life care for adults (QS13) www.nice.org.uk/guidance/qualitycarestandards/endoflifecare/home/jsp

[8] LCP Central Team. What is the Liverpool Care pathway for the Dying Patient? Information for Healthcare Professionals. www.mcpcil.org.uk (accessed June 22, 2013; no longer accessible September 2019).

guidance from the General Medical Council,[9] the Royal College of Physicians[10] and the British Medical Association.[11] Most of this guidance was available free of charge online. The pathway aimed not only to improve care in the last few hours or days of life, but also to improve knowledge related to the dying process. Research into end-of-life are presents particular challenges, but there is a need for better knowledge on patient views on dying well as well as on techniques of palliative care. Better data on how people die, as opposed to what they die of, is required.[12]

The LCP had *three key sections*: initial assessment, ongoing assessment and care after death; and *four key domains of care*: physical, psychological, social and spiritual; and *five key requirements* for organisational governance: clinical decision making, management & leadership, learning & teaching, research & development, governance and risk. Simply setting that out made it immediately apparent that using the pathway would only be as good as the teams using it. It could not be applied to the right standard without education and training.

Some of those features required emphasis in the light of recent controversy. The LCP was not designed to either hasten or prolong death and its application required good communication with all involved: patients, families and carers, professionals. Not only did it not preclude a policy of no hydration or nutrition, but it considered a blanket policy of no artificial hydration or nutrition to be unethical. It did not recommend continuous deep sedation. Continuous reassessment was a feature with a formal full multi-disciplinary team (MDT) meeting every 3 days. By law, all decisions had to be made in the patient's best interests. A properly constituted advance refusal of treatment by a patient has full legal force in the UK and cannot be overruled. The emphasis on reassessment reflected little more than the uncertainties under which all medicine is practised.[13] Prognostication is often inaccurate, especially in the dying patient. The ability for self-care, oral intake, conscious level and so on, may all change and make a review of needs essential.

2.3 The Controversy

It was against this background that from 2010 onwards a series of concerns was expressed in the UK about the use of the LCP. For example, a psychiatrist expressed concerns that artificial nutrition and hydration was not given to patients on the LCP;

---

[9] General Medical Association. Treatment and care towards the end of life. London, 2010.

[10] Royal College of Physicians of London. Oral Feeding Difficulties and dilemmas. A guide to practical care particularly towards the end of life. London, 2010.

[11] British Medical Association. Withholding and withdrawing Life-prolonging medical Treatment. Guidance for Decision making. (3rd edition). London, 2007.

[12] Royal College of Physicians of London. Research on patients at the end of life. In: Guidelines on the practice of ethics committees in medical research (4th edition). London, 2007, p66.

[13] Saunders J. Do we really have to live with this? Uncertainty in medicine. In: Philosophy in Medicine: Applications in a Clinical Context. Ed M Evans, P Louhiala, R Puustinen. Radcliffe Medical Press, Oxford, 2004, 97–110.

another consultant alleged 'backdoor euthanasia' in a major broadsheet newspaper, the *Daily Telegraph*. The *Telegraph* was joined by the *Daily Mail* and the two papers maintained a campaign of criticism against the "pathway of death". For example, in one widely publicised case, Susan Goold complained that her father had been placed on the LCP without permission and had suffered a "barbaric death" deprived of food and fluid for 8 days, without being able to say farewell to his wife and with no record in his case notes about the LCP.[14] The daughter's claim was reported that "You wouldn't treat a dog the way my poor dad was treated. We are all devastated, the best interests of the patient was not starving him to death." The hospital, Addenbrooke's in Cambridge, was left to investigate. Similar reports of this sort appeared throughout this period and the press campaign widened to further allegations. Thus the *Daily Mail* reported that "Hospitals were bribed to put patients on the pathway to death…The incentives have been paid to hospitals that ensure that a set percentage of patients who die on their wards have been put on the controversial regime. At least £ 30 million in extra money from taxpayers has been handed to hospitals in the last 3 years to achieve these goals.[15]" Addenbrooke's Hospital, involved in the Goold case, for example, had received over £1 million according to the *Daily Telegraph*. A BBC investigation reported that only 57% patients had their care plan discussed with relatives or carers. And in a story in November 2012, the *Daily Mail* ran a story on its front pages entitled "Now sick babies of on death pathway." The story claimed[16] that NHS hospitals were discharging sick children and babies to hospices or their homes, where food and fluid were withdrawn until they died. The story was based on the testimony of a doctor practising in another country, never disclosed. Further criticisms followed against a well-known UK children's hospital with as little substance. But the *Daily Mail* did not remove the story from its website or correct or clarify it. It was published in a different version in the *Daily Telegraph* and inspired scores of responses from readers expressing disgust that the NHS permitted such practice – which of course it doesn't.

A prominent *Daily Mail* columnist, Melanie Phillips, wrote rhetorically "Care?" and replied to herself, "No, this is a pathway to killing people that doctors deem useless.[17]" Further inflammatory allegations and opinions followed from Phillips' pen: "In other words, they are killed. What's more, they are killed in a most cruel and callous way through starvation and dehydration." Patrick Pullicino, a consultant neurologist and professor of clinical neurosciences at Kent University, was reported as telling a conference that the LCP had become an 'assisted death pathway' for more than 100,000 patients each year. 'Very likely, many elderly patients who could live substantially longer are being killed by the LCP,' he said. "Horrifyingly, (Phillips went on) the LCP has become a self-fulfilling prophecy. When people are

[14] Daily Mail. March 6, 2013 (Accessed online June 23, 2013).

[15] McCartney M. The assault on the Liverpool Care Pathway. BMJ 2012;345:e7316.

[16] Arie S. Inquiry launched into newspaper story about babies on "death pathway". BMJ 2013;35:e7718.

[17] Daily Mail. October 14, 2012 (Accessed online June 23, 2013).

put on it, they are said to be dying. But they may not be dying at all — not, that is, until they are put on the 'pathway', whereupon they really do die as a result.... This really is an obscene abuse of people who expect the NHS to care for them, not kill them. And how appalling that this has made patients terrified that the hospitals supposedly taking care of them may try instead to kill them." The LCP was being driven both by crude economic calculations and by a wider brutalisation of our culture at the heart of which lay the erosion of respect for the innate value of human life supported by the "lethal arrogance"[18] of the medical profession. Phillips had her sympathisers among doctors too. One wrote to the BMJ stating that she should be applauded for highlighting an area of practice that the letter writer thought "clearly" warranted investigation.[19]

2.4 The Response

There was a strong professional response. Doctors do not commonly write *en masse* to the press, but on November 6, 2012 a letter was sent to the *Daily Telegraph* signed by 1300 doctors who said that they supported the pathway. The Press Complaints Commission received 311 complaints about one of the *Daily Mail*'s article. Nevertheless, there were conflicting voices[20] even if few doctors would support the inflammatory critique advanced by Phillips. Most believed, along with a BMJ columnist, that end of life care had been transformed.[21] A group of organisations issued a consensus statement backing the LCP and reiterating that it was about excellence in care: "Published misconceptions and often inaccurate information...risk detracting from the substantial benefits it can bring to people who are dying and to their families.[22]" Those backing the statement included the Royal College of Physicians, the Royal College of General Practitioners, the British Geriatrics Society, charities, organisations representing care homes, social services, hospitals and palliative care services. It had already been pointed out that the alleged payments concerned incentives to achieve the multiple targets and frameworks used to judge hospitals' performance; these were not bribes but typical sources of income and entirely usual. Moreover conversations were happening. The perception that patients were placed on the LCP without discussion reflected the failure to name the LCP rather than a lack of description of the care being offered.

---

[18] Daily Mail 30 October 2012 (accessed online June 22, 2013).

[19] Teo I. The assault on the Liverpool Care Pathway. BMJ 2012;345:e7316 (accessed June 22, 2013).

[20] O'Dowd A. Liverpool care pathway: doctors speak out. BMJ 2012;345:e7644.

[21] Spence D. How end of life care has been transformed. BMJ 2012;35:e7308.

[22] Kmietowicz Z. Doctors leaders, charities, and hospices back Liverpool Care Pathway. BMJ 213:345:e6654.

An investigation of doctors views was carried out by the BMJ in association with the television programme *Dispatches* on Channel 4 TV.[23] This surveyed 563 doctors who had used the pathway. They comprised 185 consultants in palliative medicine, 168 in training or career grade posts in palliative medicine and 210 doctors in other specialties. The survey demonstrated widespread concern and reluctance to use the LCP due to requests from relatives or apprehension about relatives' complaints. Negative press was leading to more distress and a fear that discussion would increase those anxieties. Almost none thought that bed pressures had led to LCP use. However only 13% of respondents thought that financial incentives should be used to encourage use of the LCP. As one said, "Setting targets for the use of a tool that was intended simply to ensure best practice was never wise and always open to misinterpretation." Training needs were often not met, but the respondents were clear in pointing out that the problem was not primarily with the LCP – it was as foolish as blaming insulin for the damage and deaths it has caused due to misuse. 91% thought the LCP represented best practice and 98% thought that it allowed patients to die with dignity. 90% said they would want the pathway themselves in a terminal illness (and some of the remaining 10% may represent confusion from the use of a modified version in Welsh respondents). "Scaremongering was putting end of life care back about twenty years, where dying patients were hidden in side rooms and not seen by a consultant."

2.5 Further Considerations

Certainly it was true that the CLP should not have been used as a way to indicate that the patient's care was 'palliative' (or worse, 'patient is palliative'); or a way to ensure that appropriate medication was prescribed for patients *not* judged to be in last hours/days of life; or a way to stop clinicians thinking about that particular patients' needs, or avoid using clinical judgement; or a way to prescribe a syringe driver, for a patient being on a syringe driver does not indicate that the patient is dying or on the LCP. Whether the patient is dying in hours or days is a clinical judgement which sometimes we will get wrong and the LCP should have been discontinued if the patient's condition improved. The problem created by the press campaign was that patients, relatives, carers and some staff were worried about the LCP and many wrongly may have felt that it was 'euthanasia', or used to hasten death. There was the spectre of a belief that the LCP represented the concept of a 'pathway' to lead to death. And with successive versions, the LCP had become a large document, extended to avoid problems of earlier versions. For example, 'Variance' takes time to complete so nurses might just put 'A' for 'achieved' beside goals. If misapplied or misused due to lack of education or training that practice carried risks for patients. Already many proposals had been discussed about

[23] Chinthapalli K. The Liverpool Care Pathway: what do specialists think? BMJ 2013;346:f1184.

possible improvements. Some suggested getting rid of the terms ‘pathway’ and ‘Liverpool’; considering whether there ought to be national guidance on care and prescribing for patients imminently dying but not in ‘pathway’ format. Others suggested that there are problems with the term ‘care plan’ as the latter is particular to a patient, and the term has multiple uses. Certainly most agreed that if the LCP (or similar) was to continue, it required dedicated mandatory training, with funding, to avoid known risks of misapplication, and misuse. And financial incentives or penalties had to be removed as they plainly led to misunderstanding.

What was this heated debate about? Was it that there are fundamental problems with the LCP, despite the accolades that it has received by expert bodies? Was it improper use of the ‘pathway’, perhaps due to misapplication (to the wrong patient), or to misuse (not following it properly), arising, for example, in relation to a lack of the necessary specific training? Or was it misrepresentation and scaremongering by the media, especially the *Daily Mail* and *Daily Telegraph*? Certainly there has been evidence of patients put on the LCP without the specified MDT approval, patients who were terminally ill but not in the last few hours or days of life, and those who have not had all reversible pathologies treated. In a population of about 60 million in the UK, there are about 550,000 deaths each year. It would be surprising if every one went according to plan, noble though that aspiration may be. Probably all of these factors have played their role.

2.6 The Neuberger Inquiry

National debate led to government action – to reassure an anxious public or reform a faulty policy. An independent inquiry was set up by the health minister, Norman Lamb, under the chairmanship of Rabbi Baroness Julia Neuberger. This reported in the summer of 2013.[24] Its conclusions were mixed: the LCP, properly used, was able to deliver high quality care for the dying; on the other hand, it had not always been properly used. The group stated at the outset that, regardless of how far its recommendations were accepted, “there needs to be a proper National Conversation about dying. Otherwise doctors and nurses are likely to become the whipping-boys for an inadequate understanding of how we face our final days.” The recommendations included:

- phasing out the LCP and replacing it with an individual end of life care plan
- a general principle that a patient should only be placed on the LCP or a similar approach by a senior responsible clinician in consultation with the healthcare team
- unless there is a very good reason, a decision to withdraw or not to start a life-prolonging treatment should not be taken during any ‘out of hours’ period

[24] More Care, Less Pathway: a Review of the Liverpool Care Pathway https://www.gov.uk/government/publications/review-of-liverpool-care-pathway-for-dying-patients

- an urgent call for the Nursing and Midwifery Council to issue guidance on end of life care
- an end to incentive payments for use of the LCP and similar approaches
- a new system-wide approach to improving the quality of care for the dying.

It was stated that the term 'pathway' was clearly being misunderstood; and it was critical of the fact that *independent, prospective* testing of the LCP had not been carried out after nearly 10 years of its dissemination. The Review panel heard many instances of both good and bad decision-making; some of the latter were occurring at sub-optimal times: in the middle of the night, at weekends or on Bank Holidays. There had been concerns around consent that required addressing. Other issues covered included comment on hydration and nutrition; sedation & pain management; attempted CPR; and hastening death. The environment of care, accountability and documentation were all covered. Care of the elderly was an area with some overlap in a scandal of excess deaths in Stafford, that had led to an earlier, lengthier report[25] with widespread repercussions in British medicine. Equipment and training were also the subject of comment. The training issues were addressed and the critical comment made that "many of the problems in the care of the dying highlighted in this report are due to poor understanding among clinicians of existing guidance in care for the dying, and an unwillingness to discuss with patients, their relatives and carers the prospect of death and the clinical uncertainties that accompany it".

In May 2014, the Royal College of Physicians published a National Care of the Dying Audit[26] based on 6580 people dying in 149 hospitals between May 1 and 31, 2013. This included a case notes review of a sample; and questionnaires from 858 relatives and/or friends. Perhaps predictably, practice fell short of ideal standards of care and the report contains data and lessons of value to anyone interested in the provision of care at the end of life – not just in the UK. It might be concluded that care plans etc. are valuable tools in end of life care but only a small part. Professional shortcomings reflect a wider societal denial of death and its discussion. Addressing this needs education, training, an adequate workforce, audit and the other interventions recommended in both the Neuberger Report and the RCP Audit. But chiefly, there is the need to capture the hearts and minds of professionals in many specialties to make a commitment to this area of patient care – to understand death as an experience that requires a sensitive, informed and committed expertise. The willingness to investigate the standards of care, publish uncomfortable findings in detail and make recommendations is surely to be commended. In this, at least, the UK medical establishment can take considerable credit.

Acknowledgements I am grateful to my colleague, Dr. Fiona Randall, consultant in palliative medicine, for discussion and advice; and to Professor Pierre Mallia for the invitation to present and discuss these issues at a conference in Malta in March, 2013.

[25] Final report of the Mid Staffordshire NHS Foundation Trust Public Inquiry http://www.midstaffspublicinquiry.com/report

[26] https://www.rcplondon.ac.uk/resources/national-care-dying-audit-hospitals

A Postscript to the LCP Controversy

In June 2015, the UK's Department of Health & Social Care published an independent report ("One Chance to get it Right") on how health and social care organisations should care for people in the last days of life.[27] This followed irregularities about practice at the end of life alleged to result from misapplication of the Liverpool Care Pathway (as above). These concerns had led to the independent report and its recommendations ("More Care, Less Pathway") from a group set up under the chairmanship of Baroness Rabbi Julia Neuberger. "One Chance to get it Right" was a response to the Neuberger report's recommendations from the Leadership Alliance for the Care of Dying People, made up of 21 national health and care organisations. The Alliance's objectives were to support those involved in the care of people who are dying to respond to the findings of the Neuberger review; and be the focal point for the system's response its findings and recommendations. The Alliance's work represents a substantial contribution to improving standards of care, running to 168 pages, together with 28 pages of 'Commitment statements' and a 39 page 'Summary of engagement on proposed outcomes and guiding principles for care in the last days of life'. It incorporated comments from families and those who attended workshops set up by the Alliance, as well as online responses. It covered the new Care Quality Commission inspection regime for end of life care, new NICE guidance, actions to improve education, training and research; professional regulation; and the implementation of the priorities for care.

At around the same time, the (devolved) Welsh Assembly Government published "Together for Health – Delivering End of Life Care A Delivery Plan up to 2016 for NHS Wales and its Partners." This set up "The Wales Palliative Care Implementation Board" to provide support and scrutiny. The world's largest palliative care medical representative body, the UK and Ireland's Association for Palliative Medicine,[28] continues to issue position statements and educational material that update guidance on specific issues as they develop.

All these materials warrant study. I think it may be concluded that while many of the critical claims made over the Liverpool Care Pathway may have been exaggerated or even untrue, the effect of the controversy has been to focus minds on developing guidance that is thorough, comprehensive and practical. It offers both guidance to professionals and to all of us as we face our own mortality, the hope and prospect of the best supportive care.

[27] https://www.gov.uk/government/publications/improvements-to-care-in-the-last-days-and-hours-of-life Accessed Sept 9, 2019.

[28] https://apmonline.org/

Chapter 3
Spirituality, Religion, and Psychology

Renzo Pegoraro

Abstract Spirituality, religion and psychology have three distinct areas of applications, each one with its peculiar characteristics. Spirituality in general includes a sense of connection to something bigger than ourselves, and it typically involves a search for meaning in life. Religion is the set of beliefs, feelings, dogmas and practices that define the relations between the human being and the sacred or divine. Psychology is the study, with the methods of empirical sciences, of the functions that can be referred to the mind or the soul, i.e. cognition, emotions, motivations, personality. The chapter analyses the relation between the realms of spirituality, religion and psychology, their similarities and their differences, their methodological approaches and objects. Their relationship with health, illness and process of dying is also taken into consideration, where concepts like body, soul, beliefs, values, traditions and practices are involved. Spiritual distress may result from some serious illness situations, with its burden of suffering and pain, up to the extreme experience of death. It is very important that an approach is taken from a multidisciplinary perspective. Consequently, the actors involved will also be different, each with their own specific characteristics and objectives: patients, healthcare professionals, family and Institutions.

Keywords Spirituality · End of life · Spiritual distress · Religion · Psychology · Health

3.1 Introduction

Although spirituality, religion and psychology, may overlap in some respects, they have three distinct areas of application, each one with its peculiar characteristics.

According to social sciences, religion is the set of beliefs, feelings, dogmas and practices that define the relations between human being and sacred or divinity. Even if the definition falls short in many ways – e.g. the very important role of reason

R. Pegoraro (✉)
Pontifical Academy for Life, Vatican City, Rome, Italy
e-mail: cancelliere@pav.va

P. Mallia et al. (eds.), *Challenges to the Global Issue of End of Life Care*,
Advancing Global Bioethics 17, https://doi.org/10.1007/978-3-030-86386-9_3

(*logos*) involved in theological reflection about faith experience in many religious traditions is absent – we will refer to it as a generic and operational tool for our discourse.

A religion may be defined with its three great characteristics:

- Believes and religious practices
- The religious feeling/virtue i.e. faith
- Unity in a community of those who share the same faith.

There is a very large variety in the rites, doctrines and practices of different religions.

Religious beliefs and participation are ubiquitous within and across populations. From a global perspective, approximately 84% of the world's population report a religious affiliation: 31.5% Christianity, 23.2% Islam, 15% Hinduism, 7.1% Buddhism, 5.9% Folk religions, 0,2% Judaism, and 0.8% Other. Only 16.3% report being religiously unaffiliated.

Within the United States, 89% believe in God or a universal spirit, 78% consider religion a very important or fairly important part of life, 79% identify with a particular religious group, and 36% report having attended a religious service in the review, the associations between religious participation and health are likewise considerable in magnitude (Balboni and Peteet 2017).

Spirituality is a broad concept with room for many perspectives. In general, it includes a sense of connection to something bigger than ourselves, and it typically involves a search for meaning in life. As such, it is a universal human experience—something that touches us all. People may describe a spiritual experience as sacred or transcendent (as a religion) or simply a deep sense of aliveness and interconnectedness.

Psychology comes from Greek: "psyche". It is the word for "mind" (or "soul"), and "logos" and it means discourse. In other words, psychology is the study, with the methods of empirical sciences, of the functions that can be referred to the mind or the soul. Therefore, psychology deals with the processes of sense perception, thinking, learning, cognition, emotions and motivations, and personality, focusing on the behavior of individuals. Philosophers used to discuss many topics now studied by modern psychology, such as memory, free will, attraction etc. Such topics overlap also with spirituality and religion.

These definitions and distinctions are not always easy when considering the different religious and spiritual traditions worldwide, especially when looking at Western countries, Eastern countries and the African continent.

Here, a broad global approach has been sought, an approach that recognizes the differences, but also the commonalities that make it possible to talk about religion, spirituality, and psychology. And today, in a globalized world, there is greater interconnection and dialogue among countries, but even within the same country, at the local level. And it is important to take into account how different religions can contribute to addressing ethical end-of-life issues, supporting spiritual accompaniment in palliative care.

3.2 Spirituality Vs. Religion: A Debate with Many Connotations

Religion and spirituality are two related yet distinct terms associated with faith.

Spirituality refers to an interior dynamic of search for meaning in life, so that it is connected with an experience of the individual person.

Religion has an institutional dimension and refers to sets of truths and practices, somehow dependent on a divine revelation, that are also relevant in the public sphere and have a social impact. Even if it is not impossible to be religious without being spiritual and spiritual without being religious, the two dimensions are normally connected.

Spirituality is more abstract than religion and exists in a realm with wider borders. An increasing number of people in postmodern Western culture claim to have a spirituality without belonging to a specific religious community.

3.3 Psychology Vs Spirituality: A Sharp Divide?

Spirituality and psychology are two complex subjects to discuss and they become even more complicated when you try to relate one to the other. There is a great debate between practitioners of psychology and those of spirituality. The major difference among them is the methodological approach: the object of psychology is framed by the conceptual and practical tools that are specific of empirical sciences, while spirituality is in a broader sense referred to an existential experience. An experience that can be harbored in different context of human activities and practices. So, we can recur to both to have a deeper and non-confessional understanding of human beings in medical practice.

3.4 Religion Vs. Psychology: Room for Dialogue

The relationship between religion and psychology usually involves the study of religious belief and behavior from a psychological perspective. Throughout history, scholars and researchers have tried to identify the one key reason that people are attracted to religion. Some have said people seek religion to cope with a fear of death, others call it the basis for morality.

For many people, religion and spirituality are key resources that can facilitate their growth. For others, religion and spirituality may be sources of problems that need to be addressed in the service of their health and well-being. Some psychologists have characterized religious beliefs as pathological, seeing religion as a malignant social force that encourages irrational thoughts and ritualistic behaviors. Emerging research is showing that spiritually-integrated approaches to treatment are as effective as other psychological treatments. There are therefore good scientifically based reasons to be more sensitive to religion and spirituality in clinical practice (Balboni and Peteet 2017). Psychologists are now developing and evaluating a variety of spiritually integrated approaches to treatment.

3.5 Religion and Health

Religion is concerned with health in its broadest sense, that of wholeness or well-being. In fact, religious participation contributes to physical and mental health and subjective wellbeing, through shaping behavior, creating systems of meaning, altering one's outlook on life, building community and social support supporting moral choices for personal and societal good, and through an experience of the transcendent. Of course it cannot be overlooked that religious understanding of health, and even life, is subordinated to higher values: think of a missionary who travels in unhealthy regions where health and life are at risk in order to take care of refugees or sick people. The overall meaning of his/her life is broader than a physical one.

At the same time, it is communal forms of religious participation, rather than merely private practices, that most powerfully affect health.

Religious communities and persons can promote health through caregiving, health-promotion interventions, spiritual care in medical and end-of-life settings, forgiveness interventions, and by simply offering a form of meaningful communal participation.

A religious understanding of health, illness, and well-being, and of the actions needed to promote health, will often make appeal to theological concepts such as sin, salvation, character, love, divine action, and forgiveness (Balboni and Peteet 2017).

3.6 Religious Beliefs About Major End-of-Life Issues

Religion and spirituality are important factors that shape the way the care is provided. According to a recent position paper signed by representatives of the Abrahamic monotheistic religions (Christianity, Judaism, Islam) on matters concerning the end of life, they agree in terms of their views about major end-of life issues (Pontifical Academy for Life 2019). They advocate for the holistic and respectful care of the person which requires compassion, empathy and professionalism on the part of every person involved in the care of the patient. Any dying patient should receive the best possible comprehensive palliative care, while matters pertaining to the duration and meaning of human life should not be in the domain of health care providers. Spiritual and religious assistance is a fundamental right of the patient and a duty of the faith community.

Different religions may vary in terms of other important medical issues at the end of life. We recognize major difference between Western and Eastern religious traditions. For example, pharmacotherapy for pain control can have different implications for people belonging to different religions. The Judeo-Christian view endorses the use of pain medications as long as the intent is to comfort the dying patient. However, Eastern religions (including Hinduism and Buddhism) often object to the use of opioid medications at the end of life due to the undesirable consequence of a decreased level of consciousness at the time of death. Furthermore, end of life fasting is sometimes considered to be a source of spiritual purification by Hindus, and so they might object to tube feeding once the end is near (Setta and Shemie 2015).

Different views affect also the meaning and the way death occurs. Christianity and the other Western traditions, for example, believes that death happens when the soul leaves the body; Buddhism sees death occurring at a point after the invisible, subtle consciousness leaves the physical body. Because these events are not visible, religions turn to different empirical evidence to determine that death has occurred, shaping the ways in which their ethical analysis and decision making in the event of a terminal illness take place. The official position of the Catholic Church, for example, firmly asserts that brain death is death, there is no difficulty in ending the mechanical means that was used to support the patient prior to the determination of death. In Judaism, withdrawing mechanical support at any point is at least as controversial in the orthodox community as the criteria used to define death. Even those who favor using neurological criteria find it difficult to discontinue mechanical support, especially the ventilator, even though the patient has met the criteria for brain death. In Islam, though the issue of how to determine if someone has died remains contentious, there is little disagreement on withdrawing futile treatment. The physician and family are charged with making this decision. Factors that can be considered include the benefit to be derived from the treatment, the burden to the patient and the burden to the family. Hindu concern for both interfering with the timing of death and allowing the individual to focus correctly shows itself directly in attitudes toward suspending treatment, especially mechanical means of life support (Chakraborty et al. 2017).

However, perspectives may vary even within the same religion based on the subgroup to which the patient or provider belong, or even their country of residence. A nation's cultural practices and laws usually have a significant influence on beliefs and practices. Level of education can also play an important role. Increasing cultural competency in practitioners should include the reasoning process religions use to determine the correct approach in the face of death.

3.7 Spirituality at the End of Life

"Let no one persuade you to cure the head, until he has first given you his soul to be cured by the charm. For this is the great error of our day in the treatment of the human body, that physicians separate the soul from the body. You cannot heal one without taking care of the other." This sentence by the Greek Philosopher Socrates, illustrates very well the link between body and soul. The same link that comes into play in the relationship between spirituality and health (Coob et al. 2012).

The word «spiritual» can be ambiguous. As I already pointed out, spiritual refers to concerns about the ultimate meaning and values in life. It has to do with our deepest sense of who we are and what life is all about. 'Spiritual' does not immediately imply belief in a supreme being or in a life after this. Atheists have spiritual concerns just like everyone else.

Spirituality applies to both believers and non-believers, that in this sense should be better called 'alternative' believers.

As people are faced with serious illness or the prospect of dying, questions often arise:

- Why did this happen to me?
- What will happen to me after I die?
- Why would God allow me to suffer this way?
- Will I be remembered?
- Will I be missed?

C. Puchalski defined spirituality as "a dynamic and intrinsic aspect of humanity, through which persons seek ultimate meaning, purpose, and transcendence, and experience relationship to self, family, community… sacred (God)" (Puchalski et al. 2009). Spirituality then can also be expressed through beliefs, values, traditions and practices (Puchalski et al. 2014).

3.8 Spiritual Distress

Serious illness can rock patients' beliefs and may represent a time of profound questioning, in an attempt to search for meaning to the event, yielding spiritual distress.

According to North American Nursing Diagnosis Association (NANDA 2014), spiritual distress involves impaired ability to experience and integrate meaning and purpose in life through connectedness with self, others, art…, and/or a Power Greater than oneself. It expresses itself through grief/loss, hopelessness, conflict about beliefs, feelings of remoteness from deity/God, anger towards God, a deep existential state of suffering, and, the seeking of spiritual assistance.

In a crisis situation, the believer may turn to his/her religion for help as a source of hope and strength. The non-believer may turn to his/her inner energy or external power, such as connectedness with others or nature.

In this state, the individual is in a position to weigh and evaluate the essential significance of life and death.

When approaching death, you can go through several steps: fulfilment, leave, suffering, fear, preparing for the *vis-à-vis* meeting with God, religious dimension and rites.

Some ethical aspects may concern «living will/advanced directives», proxy/tutor, problem of pain and suffering, avoidance of therapeutic obstinacy, euthanasia, palliative care, and, Advanced Care Planning (Best et al. 2020).

3.9 Regarding a Spiritual Dimension

(a) *Responsibility of the patient.*

Regarding the spiritual dimension, the responsibility of the patient himself/herself has to do with the recognition of this personal dimension, but also to find the meaning of this condition and crises, to «draw off» from the personal biography and history of hope, faith, spiritual experiences, to the seeking of spiritual assistance.

(b) *The Health Care Professionals.*

The Health Care Professionals should be able to take care of their own spirituality in order to be able to recognize that of others and to provide a meaningful experience of "humanity". They should favor an interprofessional and interdisciplinary approach, get in involved a deep and genuine relationship with the sick person, retrieve and integrate a unitary-holistic view of the person, highlight the "spiritual need" and be able to choose "competent" people for this (Best et al. 2020).

It is important to define models of diagnosis of spiritual distress at the generalist approach and the specialist one, and a specialist professional should be available (chaplain, rabbi, imam, spiritual counsellor…) in a multiethnic and multireligious context through listening, dialogue, sensitivity, specific training and adequate knowledge (Best et al. 2020).

3.10 Helping and Assisting Until the End

(a) *Patient not in solitude*

The patient should not be left alone with his fears, his anxieties, his doubts about the disease, the diagnosis, the prognosis.

The relationship with the patient cannot have an expiry date but must be prolonged, constant, tending towards the truth, assuring continuity of care and assistance, attending to suffering: being present through a welcoming listening.

The so-called "spiritual hospitality" is the gift of presence and accompanying, that are the hallmarks of Palliative care and spiritual support.

All subjects linked to the patients should have a role in this; family members, caregivers, health care workers, volunteers, chaplains. etc.

(b) *Healthcare Professionals.*

As far as health care professional workers are concerned, they should be able to work in teams of different professionals to ensure this holistic approach. It is important to take care of the "spirit of the team", to encourage communication as far as possible, to share feelings, hopes, disappointments. And to pay attention to defense mechanisms and the risks of "burn-out "and/or "moral distress" for the professionals themselves. One should guard against forms of "sentimentalism" or "magic" or "spiritualism", ensuring professionality and specificity of one's own role (Perkins 2016).

(c) *The family*

We cannot but also consider the impact of the terminal ill patient on the family and the crucial role of the family as caregiver. So spiritual support must not only be offered to the patient but to the members of the family as well.

(d) *Institutions*

Institutions, therefore, should recognize the importance of spirituality and strive for its integration in care and palliative care, realizing appropriate social responses, helping to develop the spiritual dimension of care and implement organizational measures to facilitate personal and communitarian "rites". In other words, helping "to live" until the end and to accompany the patient in preparation of a "good death" (Foley 2018).

It is becoming more and more relevant and urgent to support initiatives of high quality, multidisciplinary academically accessible spiritual care education to all palliative care staffs.

A multidisciplinary education is very important encouraging, the development, the skill of self-reflection for the healthcare professional involved in palliative care and a holistic approach to the patients, including screening for spiritual needs and supporting spiritual care (Sulmasy 2002; Best et al. 2020).

3.11 Conclusion

The spiritual dimension of health care may often be omitted in many settings or provided simply by having a spiritual counsellor available who may, especially in large institutions, not have enough time to spend with the dying patient besides a few moment and to give some form of special rite towards the end. It is seen here how spirituality is not only about religious rites but forms a holistic component considered very important at the end of life both for the patient and for the family. This give a more meaningful end for all those concerned – patient, family and the health care professionals themselves.

With an attentive look at globalization and the interactions between various religions also at a global and local level, it is possible to see how adequate palliative care can include and develop adequate spiritual care, with personalized responses to individual patients and families, with their religious faiths and spiritual needs.

Different religious traditions can play an important role in a holistic approach to the sick person, with attention to spiritual distress, in order to elaborate a good accompaniment in the final stages of life (Carrasco de Paula and Pegoraro 2015).

A sincere dialogue and effective collaboration among all these domains, i.e. religion, spirituality and psychology, involving these different care professionals, can help to promote a person-centered approach, supporting the patients and families in the dying process. And this approach helps the health care team in its "spirit" of caring, compassion, human experience at the bedside of terminal hill patients (Benton and Pegoraro 2021).

References

Balboni, M., and J. Peteet, eds. 2017. *Spirituality and religion within the culture of medicine*. Oxford: Oxford University Press.

Benton, K., and R. Pegoraro. 2021. *Finding dignity at the end of life. A spiritual reflection on palliative care*. New York: Routledge.

Best, M., et al. 2020. An EAPC white paper on multi-disciplinary education for spiritual care in palliative care. *BMC Palliative Care* 19: 9. https://doi.org/10.1186/s12904-019-0508-4.

Carrasco De Paula, I., and R. Pegoraro, eds. 2015. *Assisting the elderly and palliative care*. Rome: Pontifical Academy for Life.

Chakraborty, R., A. El-Jawahri, M.R. Litzow, et al. 2017. A systematic review of religious beliefs about major end-of-life issues in the five major world religions. *Palliative & Supportive Care* 15 (5): 609–622.

Coob, M.R., C.M. Puchalski, and B. Rumbold, eds. 2012. *Oxford textbook of spirituality in healthcare*. Oxford: Oxford University Press.

Foley, M. 2018. Accompanying life in the passage of death. In *Accompanying life. New Responsabilities in the technological era*, ed. V. Paglia and R. Pegoraro. Rome: Pontifical Academy for Life.

NANDA International. 2014. In *Nursing diagnoses: Definitions and classification 2015-2017*, ed. T.H. Herdman and S. Kamitsuru. Oxford: Wiley Blackwell.

Perkins, H. 2016. *A guide to psychosocial and spiritual Care at the end of life*. New York: Springer.

Pontifical Academy for Life. 2019, October 28. *Position paper on the Abrahamic Monoteistic Religions on matters concerning the end of life*. Vatican City.

Puchalski, C.M., B. Ferrel, et al. 2009. Improving the quality of spiritual care as a dimension of palliative care. *J. Pall. Med* 12: 885–904.

Puchalski, C.M., R. Vitillo, S.K. Hull, and N. Reller. 2014. Improving the spiritual dimension of whole person care: Reaching national and international consensus. *J. Pall. Med.* 14: 642–656.

Setta, S.M., and S.D. Shemie. 2015. An explanation and analysis of how world religions formulate their ethical decisions on withdrawing treatment and determining death. *Philosophy, Ethics, and Humanities in Medicine* 10: 6. https://doi.org/10.1186/s13010-015-0025-x.

Sulmasy, D. 2002. A biopsycho-social-spiritual model for the care of patients at the end of life. *Gerontologist* 42: 24–33.

Chapter 4
Global Systems: Palliative Care and Hospices at the End of Life

Piret Paal

Anyway, if you stopped tellin' people it's all sorted out after they're dead, they might try sorting it all out while they're alive.

Terry Pratchett, Good Omens

Abstract Inability to address health-related suffering that initially descends from universal death-denial is an informal political endorsement for futile treatments and a human rights violation. This chapter introduces the ethical and value-based changes in palliative care philosophy and describes the global endeavours to make palliative care available and accessible across healthcare settings. Integrated palliative care services reduce health-related suffering in all people suffering from life-limiting conditions, such as AIDS, tuberculosis (TB), comorbidities, mental ill heal, or old age frailty. This chapter argues that misconceptions, lack of education, and reluctance to develop integrated palliative care services at the country-level impede global endeavours.

Keywords Palliative care · Human rights · Health-related suffering · Universal health coverage · Education

4.1 Prologue

In his book "The Greatest Benefit to the Mankind" Porter writes: "The 'sick man' is said to have disappeared from the 'medical gaze' with the birth of the clinic around 1800, being reduced to a patient, a pathological body studded with lesions. That

---

P. Paal (✉)
WHO Collaborating Centre at the Institute of Nursing Science and Practice, Paracelsus Medical University, Salzburg, Austria
e-mail: piret.paal@pmu.ac.at

P. Mallia et al. (eds.), *Challenges to the Global Issue of End of Life Care*, Advancing Global Bioethics 17, https://doi.org/10.1007/978-3-030-86386-9_4

disappearing act continued during the next two centuries, reducing the patient in due course to an X factor in equations dominated by economics, sociology, diagnostic technology, systems analysis and multitudes of other reference frames." (Porter 1999) (page 668). Discussing the relationship between death, medicine and the people Porter continues: "From the 1960s public disquiet also grow over the depersonalisation of death within the hospital. Institutional death was viewed in the medical profession as a case of failure; the modern hospital was dedicated to saving lives, not managing death. Medicine strove to develop high-tech machinery and the protocols to accompany it, the aim being prolongation of life at all costs." (Porter 1999) (page 699). From these developments, the following three movements arose: 1. Kübler-Ross began with her death awareness movement; 2. Saunders developed an *ars moriendi* model maintaining pain relief through ample dosing of with morphine; and 3. Dutch medical society accepted euthanasia under strictly controlled circumstances in 1984 (Porter 1999) (pages 699–700). Today, all these quests are referred to as palliative care, a source of much confusion, albeit throughout the history of palliative care, its principal quest has been "to use medical measures to ease or palliate the symptoms of critically ill and dying people, combined with personalized and respectful caring." (Vanderpool 2015) (page 1).

During the twenty-first century, palliative care has gained numerous new dimensions, which are far from easing the symptoms of dying people in hospice care. Palliative care units or beds have become standard armament of modern clinics. Advanced care planning or simpler 'letters to doctors' have been widely introduced to avoid aggressive life-prolonging medical measures (Jimenez et al. 2018). Complex symptom assessment means superseding the onedimensional pain assessment (Bosnjak et al. 2011; Cherny et al. 2013; Cleary et al. 2013; Knaul et al. 2018; Lohman and Amon 2015). Access to palliative care and pain relief has is considered a human right (Lohman and Amon 2015; Radbruch et al. 2013). Palliative care is on a quest to make the 'sick man', but even more so 'the sick child' and 'the sick woman', to reappear into the 'medical gaze', and accordingly, anyone providing healthcare services should be familiar with palliative care philosophy, and able to provide it on generalist level (Paal et al. 2019). Unfortunately, the possibility that palliative care could be provided in parallel to curative therapies, or furthermore, integrated to care plan soon after diagnosing the life-threatening condition, is far from being a common understanding and practice even if evidence at hand suggests that besides improving the quality of life, palliative therapies may have a positive impact on the course of illness.

Palliative care philosophy states that palliative care provision is person-cantered and thus, based on individual needs and symptoms and not limited by prognostics. As a global ambition, palliative care is provided to all people with chronic and life-limiting conditions. This entails providing support and care for patients, young and old, as well as their informal caregivers (WHO 2018). For the latter, palliative care provides a variety of counselling services, support in bereavement and grief management. The Worldwide Palliative Care Alliance has recommended all governments to "integrate palliative care into their country's health system, alongside curative care. At a minimum, palliative care should be provided even when curative care is unavailable" (WPCA 2014) (page 8). The shift to integrated services has had a major impact on the global palliative care policy-making making it difficult for governments, service providers and educators to keep up.

This chapter introduces global strivings towards integrated palliative care as well as the new consensus based definition of palliative care. It discusses why hospices and palliative care units or beds are not enough and looks at the new global challenge, known as complex dying. Finally, the chapter refers to various policies that have been launched to improve access to integrated palliative care services globally.

4.2 Palliative Care Definition – New Features

According to WHO's palliative care definition: "Palliative care is an approach that improves the quality of life of patients and their families facing the problem associated with lifethreatening illness, through the prevention and relief of suffering by means of early identification and impeccable assessment and treatment of pain and other problems, physical, psychosocial and spiritual." (Sepúlveda et al. 2002). Palliative care for children represents a special, albeit closely related field to adult palliative care (WHO 1998). In recent years, WHO and other key stakeholders have actively worked towards awareness raising to make palliative care accessible across the globe. Therefore, it can be argued that palliative care has become a philosophy, which besides accepting death as a natural part of human life, points out the importance of collaboration between the healthcare and social sectors. This to cover the high demand for medical, social and spiritual support to guarantee continuous care, and assure patient's and informal caregivers' safety and well-being.

Close cooperation between healthcare system and social services is crucial in palliative care as often, the health and social sectors need to interact flexibly and quickly to meet the needs of the patient and family (Kaasa et al. 2018). The global success within the framework of universal health coverage, however, depends on several other factors, such as high-quality research, education, support of philanthropists and governments, as well as up to date policies and definitions. Accordingly, the International Association for Hospice and Palliative Care (IAHPC) has argued that "the current WHO definition [---] poses many challenges, limits palliative care to problems associated with life-threatening illnesses, rather than the need of patients with severe, chronic and complex conditions." (De Lima and Radbruch 2018) The mission of IAHPC has been to increase the availability and access to high quality hospice and palliative care for patients and families throughout the world (De Lima et al. 2003). Respectively, in early 2019, the IAHPC launched a new consensus based definition that approved by 400 IAHPC members from 88 countries. This definition states:

> "Palliative care is the active holistic care of individuals across all ages with serious health-related suffering due to severe illness, and especially of those near the end of life. It aims to improve the quality of life of patients, their families and their caregivers." (Radbruch et al. 2020).

Like the WHO definition from 2002, the 2019 definition clarifies different tasks of integrated palliative care. Accordingly, palliative care:

- Includes, prevention, early identification, comprehensive assessment and management of physical issues, including pain and other distressing symptoms, psychological distress, spiritual distress and social needs. Whenever possible, these interventions must be evidence based.
- Provides support to help patients live as fully as possible until death by facilitating effective communication, helping them and their families determine goals of care.
- Is applicable throughout the course of an illness, according to the patient's needs.
- Is provided in conjunction with disease modifying therapies whenever needed.
- May positively influence the course of illness.
- Intends neither to hasten nor postpone death, affirms life, and recognizes dying as a natural process.
- Provides support to the family and the caregivers during the patient's illness, and in their own bereavement.
- Is delivered recognizing and respecting the cultural values and beliefs of the patient and the family.
- Is applicable throughout all health care settings (place of residence and institutions) and in all levels (primary to tertiary).
- Can be provided by professionals with basic palliative care training.
- Requires specialist palliative care with a multiprofessional team for referral of complex cases.

The list of tasks is similar to the results of EAPC survey on post-graduate palliative care education conducted in 2018. The study indicated that when it comes to palliative care all health care providers have to (1) comprehend the palliative care philosophy; (2) be able to demonstrate the complex symptom assessment and management competencies; (3) be able to design care plans based on patients and families wishes integrating multi-professional and interdisciplinary approaches; and (4) be able to listen and self-reflect (Paal et al. 2019).

An innovative part of IAHPC's consensus definition is the to-do list for the governments. The new consensus definition suggests that to achieve palliative care integration governments should:

- Adopt adequate policies and norms that include palliative care in health laws, national health programs and national health budgets;
- Ensure that insurance plans integrate palliative care as a component of programs;
- Ensure access to essential medicines and technologies for pain relief and palliative care, including pediatric formulations;
- Ensure that palliative care is part of all health services (from community health-based programs to hospitals), that everyone is assessed, and that all staff can provide basic palliative care with specialist teams available for referral and consultation;

- Ensure access to adequate palliative care for vulnerable groups, including children and older persons;
- Engage with universities, academia and teaching hospitals to include palliative care research as well as palliative care training as an integral component of ongoing education, including basic, intermediate, specialist, and continuing education.

Getting governments to invest into palliative care is a challenge. A recent survey showed that a minority (37%) of countries have an operational national policy including palliative care. In comparison to other core service, palliative care is the least likely to have funding available. Furthermore, there is a large country-income gradient for palliative care funding, oral morphine availability, and integration of palliative care services at the primary levels of the health system (Sharkey et al. 2018). Recently published "EAPC Atlas of Palliative Care" demonstrated that 12 out of 54 European countries have systems to identify patients needing palliative care during primary care. Ten nations integrate the service early in their oncology departments; eight in cardiology, and 14 in long-term care facilities. Researchers involved in the project stress the importance of training as only 13 countries provide compulsory palliative care teaching to more than half of medical students and nine to more than 50% of nursing students. In the vast majority of Western Europe, palliative medicine is recognized as a specialty, subspecialty or specific skill area (Arias et al. 2019), which indicates a burning need for adequate national health programmes, which besides many other to-do things, include palliative care training as an integral component of ongoing education at all levels.

Of course, it is debatable whether there was a need for a new definition considering the short timeframe since the introduction of the first WHO palliative care definition. On the other hand, WHO has removed itself from its own definition in several occasions during the past years (WHO 2018; WPCA 2014). The United Nations (UN) and the World Health Organisation (WHO) have made a statement that providing access to "palliative care is an ethical responsibility of health care systems, and that it is the ethical duty of health care professionals to alleviate pain and suffering, whether physical, psychosocial or spiritual, irrespective of whether the disease or condition can be cured, and that end-of-life care for individuals is among the critical components of palliative care." (WHO 2014). "The Global Atlas of Palliative Care" states that "better, and earlier, integration of palliative care alongside active treatment is needed" (WPCA 2014) (page 8). Hence, the provision of palliative care is not limited to any care setting or certain point during the illness course. This is an integral part of Sustainable Development Goal 3 to ensure healthy lives and promote well-being for all at all ages (Powell et al. 2015). The Astana Declaration from 2018 adds that "promotive, preventive, curative, rehabilitative services and palliative care must be accessible to all." (UNICEF 2018). These global policies indicate that the understanding of palliative care philosophy is evolving, and therefore, the WHO definition from 2002 might be outdated.

4.3 Palliative Care as an Integrated Service

Historically, the modern hospice envisioned by Saunders was to provide food, lodging, personalized care and spiritual succour to patients who were frail, chronically ill, and dying, and could not be taken care at home (Vanderpool 2015) (page 127). Saunders professionalised and medicalised the hospice services. Her ultimate goal was to relieve pain and other distress, so that her patients could live more and suffer less. Until today addressing and reducing bio-psycho-social and spiritual suffering at the end of life has remained the main goal of palliative care. Without doubt, hospices and specialised palliative care teams with high ratio of staff are able to facilitate deaths in a more personalised manner than a districts nurse, GP, or most of the long-term care facilities. Specialist palliative care with a multi-professional team, however, is merely for consultations or/and referrals in complex cases.

Saunders developed her *ars moriendi* model solely as a service for terminally ill cancer patients. Accordingly, until today hospice care is the best fit for cancer patients. Modern hospices take on patients expected to die in six (or even three) months. For patients with conditions, such as old age frailty, heart failure, neurodegenerative illnesses, or multiple chronic conditions the obligation to die in a given timeframe can cause a major distress.

Although cancer death trajectories are relatively well studied and foreseeable (Sercu et al. 2018), cancer patients surviving hospices has also become a problem. Across the world, patients outlive the hospice service. Undeniably, modern palliative care can influence the course of illness in a way that a growing number of patients with complex palliative care needs end up in long-term care facilities.

Saunders' hospice was to create a 'home-like environment' for the final days of life. Moving the care from clinics to patients' homes is welcomed by many healthcare stakeholders and governments (Landers et al. 2016) due to substantially lower care costs (Kato and Fukuda 2017; Maetens et al. 2018). For patients and their families the quest 'to die at home' has become another distressful obligation. Prolonged deaths are emotionally and physically demanding for patients and informal caregivers (Boyd 2016; Duimering et al. 2017; Freeman et al. 2016; Poort et al. 2016; Uceda-Torres et al. 2016). The burden and powerlessness may even lead to violence (Pot et al. 1996; Beach et al. 2005). For formal care providers, such as GP's or nurses working at patients' homes, combining healthcare and social support needs can create barriers that healthcare providers may not be trained to navigate. In their quest to provide humanistic care to dying patients and their relatives, home care workers often face their limits (Beck et al. 2018; Arnaert et al. 2009), resulting in burnout and high turnover (Chipp et al. 2011). This is a serious problem not only in rural setting where formal care providers typically work alone but also in cities, where a growing number of sick, old and fragile people are living in unbearable conditions: often as a result of a prolonged illness trajectory and economic distress. Even if tele-health services might relieve some of the care burden (Davies et al. 2020), for many, home is not a safe place to die. Furthermore, palliative care movement is to solve questions like, how to provide 'homelike environment' to homeless people (Klop et al. 2018; Håkanson et al. 2015), prisoners (Turner and Peacock 2017; Marti et al. 2017) or asylum seekers, refugees, and vulnerable migrants (McDonald 2017; Luyirika and Enarson 2017; Roider-Schur et al. 2019). Hence, 'home-like environment' is less about home and more about safety and peace of mind, which is certainly an aspect that palliative care policy makers and governments must assess more thoroughly.

The Prague Charter of 2013 urged governments worldwide to focus efforts into developing or improving palliative care, including improving patient access to pain medication (Radbruch et al. 2013). This document was to guarantee palliative care (and pain relief) equally to AIDS patients in sub-Saharan Africa, younger people with life-limiting disease or disability, elderly people with complex care needs (Seymour 2011; Chen et al. 2010; Cibart 2010; Israels et al. 2010). Although access to palliative care and pain relief is closely monitored by Human Rights Watch (HRW 2019), the majority of governments have been reluctant to invest into high quality end-of-life care. The humanitarian effort promoted by Saunders comes with a socio-economical side, which cannot be underestimated (Scott 1994).

Hospices across the world have been and still are largely dependent on church related donors and private beneficiaries. In very few countries hospice costs are covered by insurance companies or supported by national healthcare systems. Therefore, it has been estimated that only 14% of patients have access to palliative care (and pain relief) services worldwide. When it comes to religious institutions, societal shift towards multi-faith and post-religious communities means that people are not entitled, aware of, or interested in church-related care services. This means that more locally-grown multi-faith communitybased services combining health and social services must be established to reduce the burden of all involved (Murray et al. 2015).

Saunders provided pain relief through ample dosing of with morphine. Across the globe, patients are still sent home with words: "there is nothing more we can do for you". Hence, "many patients die in severe pain within the four walls of their home; resulting people scratching the concrete walls or cracking their head because of pain" (personal communication, Bhutan 2018). Countries without access to pain medication plainly fail to meet the human right convention (Ntizimira et al. 2014; Macpherson et al. 2014; Maurer et al. 2013; Bosnjak et al. 2011; Powell et al. 2010; Brown 2004). In 2018, our WHO collaborating centre in Salzburg conducted a research travel to Central-Asia, Eastern Europe and Southeastern Europe. This fieldwork demonstrated that the imprint of 'opiophobia' is still very strong in patients and doctors, who are scared of appointing narcotic analgetics.

Patients are expected to accept pain as a final trial and physicians are afraid to prescribe. In Armenia, for example, prescribing strong opioids was sanctioned by police until recently, which meant that the prescribers ended up in prison.

Despite many global improvements, a great number of palliative care pioneers feel that politicians and national governments have not understood the importance of integrated palliative care services, which according to WHO is "a crucial part of integrated, peoplecentered health services at all levels of care" that "aims to relieve suffering, whether its cause is cancer, major organ failure, drug-resistant tuberculosis, end-stage chronic illness, extreme birth prematurity or extreme frailty of old age." (WHO 2018). Specialist services, such as hospice care or palliative care teams, are accessible only to a very limited number of patients. Despite the growing number of hospices and palliative care units, poor people and people living in areas where healthcare services are not accessible still live and die with little or no palliative care or symptom relief (Knaul et al. 2018; Krakauer et al. 2015; Krakauer et al. 2018; Kumar 2013; Lim 2008; Macpherson et al. 2014; Ntizimira et al. 2014; Powell et al. 2010; Reville and Foxwell 2014; Robinson et al. 2016). Being relocated to hospice or sent home to 'be cared, not cured' by a specially trained palliative care team is not a sustainable part of universal health coverage model aiming to guarantee quality care for all (Knaul et al. 2018; Macdonald et al. 2019).

4.4 Complex Deaths: A New Global Challenge

The global system analysis indicates that despite united efforts of multiple stakeholders and several improvements in national healthcare systems, there is a continuous rise in the burden of disease. Chang and colleagues identified 92 diseases as age related, accounting for more than half of all global burden among adults in 2017 (Chang et al. 2019). By 2030, besides the ischemic, cerebrovascular disease, lower respiratory infections, TB and AIDS, the most drastic rise has been predicted for chronic conditions, such as diabetes mellitus, stomach cancer, kidney disease and liver cancer (Mathers and Loncar 2006). People at all ages face rising levels of mental health problems and social inequities, including those linked to poverty and gender, which shape all aspects of people's health and wellbeing (Bone et al. 2018). A study conducted by Sleeman et al. (2019) estimated the global burden of diseases leading to the estimated death of 48 million people each year by 2060 (Sleeman et al. 2019). Accordingly, 130,000 people worldwide will die from serious health-related suffering each day (Chang et al. 2019).

It has been predicted that deaths will become more complex (Bone et al. 2018) and thus, more care and cost intensive. Forecasting the future global challenges, researchers have implied that healthcare and social services have to be ready to face complex and prolonged disease trajectories caused by organ failure, neurological problems (Wilson et al. 2019; Lex et al. 2018), such as mental distress, Parkinson's disease or dementia, as well as frailty (Kingston et al. 2018). All this because of the global population shift towards older adults, which is projected to rise to 16% by 2050, with the segment ages 85 and older growing the fastest (PRB 2018). Data at hand indicates that a growing number of patients with complex care needs, such as adults with severe learning disabilities, mental illness, or fragile elderly will end up in long-term care facilities (Cable-Williams and Wilson 2012; Ersek and Carpenter 2013; Lex et al. 2018). However, the implications of prolonged disease trajectories and the growing need for long-term palliative care services are rarely discussed.

A systematic review conducted in 2013 demonstrated that compared to other settings in long-term care facilities the "per person and national expenditures are notably high and these costs are highest in the last months of life, often for care that is unhelpful and unwanted" (Cable-Williams and Wilson 2012). A more recent retrospective study concluded that "elderly patients from long-term care facilities presenting with severe acute illness have high mortality and seldom receive early palliative care. The introduction of palliative care has the ability to change the course of treatment in this vulnerable population and should be considered early in the hospitalization and, where available, be initiated in the emergency department." (Mogul et al. 2019).

In England, the number of admissions in the year before death has been on the rise. If the rate continues to increase, the number of admissions will be twice as high in 2041 (Bone et al. 2018). In Germany, many long-term care facilities are critically understaffed or/and lack skilled personnel, hence, many dying patients are transferred to emergency care "just to be safe". An explorative study conducted few years ago demonstrated the lack of resources, mentors and education, which all affect the quality of care provision. Like in home care setting, many formal care providers feel trapped between the overall long-term care and end-of-life care standards (Bükki et al. 2016). Based on recent publications can be concluded that across the world staff preparedness to provide palliative care is inadequate for residents living in long-term care homes (Kaasalainen et al. 2018; Jonathan et al. 2018; Hill et al. 2018; Chan et al. 2018; Sussman et al. 2017). To address this burning issue, a European Union funded project PACE was launched in 2014 to assist long term-care facilities in making evidence-based decisions on optimal palliative care delivery to achieve the objectives of the European 2020 Strategy (Smets et al. 2018; Payne et al. 2018; Aarendonk 2014). Expectantly, the results will provide evidence based care models for long-term care facilities. Until now, introducing palliative care consult (Comart et al. 2013; Albanese et al. 2013), promoting palliative care leadership (Jonathan et al. 2018), integrating advanced care planning, such as decisions about interventions, artificial nutrition and hydration, hospitalization, antibiotics, and comfort measures (Strachan et al. 2016; Cable-Williams and Wilson 2012) has improved palliative care provision in long-term care settings. Moreover, nurses and allied healthcare professionals working in long-term care facilities need continuous support and empowerment. Such support can be provided via educational programmes, even if in many countries the availability and accessibility of palliative care education still depends solely on efforts of single pioneers. Another opportunity is to build sustainable networks with local palliative care specialists and hospices. Equally, tele-health services have proven beneficial to improve the quality of care (Weck et al. 2019).

The high number of hospital admissions and many unnecessary treatments will remain a challenge for healthcare providers in global north, whereas many low- and middle-income countries will struggle with introducing long-term care services as a culturally acceptable solution for elderly care. The major challenge for global policy making is that even among countries with similar age-standardized death rates, large differences in the onset and patterns of accumulating age-related burden exist (Chang et al. 2019). This means that the need for integrated palliative care will keep growing across the world, but governments need country and/or even community level plans to face this challenge.

4.5 Conclusion

Palliative care will continue to be a global death awareness movement and an aspirational *ars moriendi* model. Moving from specialist hospice and palliative care to integrated services is to reduce suffering and provide high quality of care for those with life-limiting illnesses across the illness trajectory. Accordingly, this chapter demonstrates that in recent years palliative care has become many things: a global movement, a care philosophy, a human right issue, and hence, challenging all healthcare providers in different settings in various ways. Globally, it is expected that a growing number people will get access to palliative care services across the field of healthcare. Equally to other global health challenges, good endof-life care and its provision need to be defined according to the local needs and resources. Therefore, it is difficult to estimate what kind of knowledge and skills healthcare professionals need to have. For example, in aging societies complex deaths are predicted to cause many care and cost intensive interventions. Nevertheless, global awareness of integrated palliative care and its benefits can help patients and their families as well as reduce the burden among healthcare provides. Currently, countries'/ governments' reluctance to invest in palliative care education and services remains the main challenge. Such insufficiency is an unofficial political endorsement for futile treatments and deathdenial.

References

Aarendonk, D. 2014. EFPC: European Forum For Primary Care comparing effectiveness of palliative care for elderly people in long-term care facilities in Europe (PACE). *European Journal of General Practice* 20: 156–156.

Albanese, T., S. Radwany, E. Hoiles, C. Hudak, and K. Mcgranahan. 2013. Building a palliative care consult service in long-term care facilities: Strategy, business model, and outcomes. *Journal of Pain and Symptom Management* 45: 418–418.

Arias, N., E. Garralda, J.Y. Rhee, and E. Al. 2019. *EAPC atlas of palliative Care in Europe 2019*. Vilvoorde: EAPC Press.

Arnaert, A., R. Seller, and M. Wainwright. 2009. Homecare nurses' attitudes toward palliative care in a rural community in Western Quebec. *Journal of Hospice & Palliative Nursing* 11: 202–208.

Beach, S.R., R. Schulz, G.M. Williamson, L.S. Miller, M.F. Weiner, and C.E. Lance. 2005. Risk factors for potentially harmful informal caregiver behavior. *Journal of the American Geriatrics Society* 53: 255–261.

Beck, I., C. Pålsson, and A.B. Tops. 2018. Upholding an ideal image of palliative work in the face of obstacles. *International Journal of Palliative Nursing* 24: 611–617.

Bone, A.E., C.J. Evans, and I.J. Higginson. 2018. The future of end-of-life care. *The Lancet* 392: 915–916.

Bosnjak, S., M.A. Maurer, K.M. Ryan, M.X. Leon, and G. Madiye. 2011. Improving the availability and accessibility of opioids for the treatment of pain: The international pain policy fellowship. *Support Care Cancer* 19: 1239–1247.

Boyd, M. 2016. My life, my death: The voices of palliative patients, informal caregivers and health care providers. *Journal of Pain and Symptom Management* 52: E95–E96.

Brown, H. 2004. WHO puts cancer on global health agenda. *The Lancet Oncology* 5: 644.

Bükki, J., P.M. Neuhaus, and P. Paal. 2016. End of life care in nursing homes: Translating focus group findings into action. *Geriatric Nursing* 37: 440–445.

Cable-Williams, B., and D.M. Wilson. 2012. Dying and palliative care of the oldest-old in long-term care facilities: Findings of an audit of decedents' records. *Journal of Palliative Care* 28: 227.

Chan, H.Y.L., G.K.M. Chun, C.W. Man, and E.M.F. Leung. 2018. Staff preparedness for providing palliative and end-of-life care in long-term care homes: Instrument development and validation. *Geriatrics & Gerontology International* 18: 745–749.

Chang, A.Y., V.F. Skirbekk, S. Tyrovolas, N.J. Kassebaum, and J.L. Dieleman. 2019. Measuring population ageing: An analysis of the global burden of disease study 2017. *The Lancet Public Health* 4: e159–e167.

Chen, Z., J. Yu, Y. Song, and D. Chui. 2010. Aging Beijing: Challenges and strategies of health care for the elderly. *Ageing Research Reviews* 9 (Suppl 1): S2–S5.

Cherny, N.I., J. Cleary, W. Scholten, L. Radbruch, and J. Torode. 2013. The Global Opioid Policy Initiative (GOPI) project to evaluate the availability and accessibility of opioids for the management of cancer pain in Africa, Asia, Latin America and the Caribbean, and the Middle East: Introduction and methodology. *Annals of Oncology* 24 (Suppl 11): xi7-13.

Chipp, C., S. Dewane, C. Brems, M.E. Johnson, T.D. Warner, and L.W. Roberts. 2011. "If only someone had told me…": Lessons from rural providers. *The Journal of Rural Health* 27: 122–130.

Cibart, J. 2010. Getting the message out about HIV/AIDS. Interview by Brenda Missen. *The Canadian Nurse* 106: 30–31.

Cleary, J., L. Radbruch, J. Torode, and N.I. Cherny. 2013. Next steps in access and availability of opioids for the treatment of cancer pain: Reaching the tipping point? *Annals of Oncology* 24 (Suppl 11): xi60-4.

Comart, J., A. Mahler, R. Schreiber, C. Rockett, R.N. Jones, and J.N. Morris. 2013. Palliative care for long-term care residents: Effect on clinical outcomes. *Gerontologist* 53: 874–880.

Connor, S.R. and Sepulveda Bermedo, M.C. 2014. *Global atlas of palliative care at the end of life*. Worldwide Hospice Palliative Care Alliance, World Health Organization. Available at Global Atlas of Palliative Care at the End of Life (thewhpca.org).

Davies, N., S. Iliffe, J. Hopwood, N. Walker, J. Ross, G. Rait, and K. Walters. 2020. The key aspects of online support that older family carers of people with dementia want at the end of life: A qualitative study. *Aging & Mental Health* 24 (10): 1654–1661. https://doi.org/10.1080/13607863.2019.1642299.

de Lima, L., and L. Radbruch. 2018. The international association for hospice and palliative care: Advancing hospice and palliative care worldwide. *Journal of Pain and Symptom Management* 55: S96–S103.

de Lima, L., E. Bruera, and R. Woodruff. 2003. The International Association for Hospice and Palliative Care: International activities and future initiatives. *Journal of Pain & Palliative Care Pharmacotherapy* 17: 31–37.

Duimering, A., J. Turner, K.P.M. Chu, F. Huang, D.M. Severin, S. Ghosh, D. Yee, E.M. Wiebe, N.H. Usmani, Z. Gabos, S.I. Patel, B. Danielson, J. Amanie, W. Roa, and A.M. Fairchild. 2017. Informal caregiver quality of life in a palliative oncology population. *International Journal of Radiation Oncology Biology Physics* 99: S87–S88.

Ersek, M., and J.G. Carpenter. 2013. Geriatric palliative care in long-term care settings with a focus on nursing homes. *Journal of Palliative Medicine* 16: 1180–1187.

Freeman, S., J.P. Hirdes, P. Stolee, and J. Garcia. 2016. A cross-sectional examination of the association between dyspnea and distress as experienced by palliative home care clients and their informal caregivers. *Journal of Social Work in End-of-Life & Palliative Care* 12: 82103.

Håkanson, C., J. Sandberg, M. Ekstedt, E. Kenne Sarenmalm, M. Christiansen, and J. Öhlén. 2015. Providing palliative care in a Swedish support home for people who are homeless. *Qualitative Health Research* 26: 1252–1262.

Hill, E., M.Y. Savundranayagam, A. Zecevic, and M. Kloseck. 2018. Staff perspectives of barriers to access and delivery of palliative Care for Persons with Dementia in long-term care. *American Journal of Alzheimers Disease and Other Dementias* 33: 284–291.

HRW. 2019. *Palliative care* [Online]. Available: https://www.hrw.org/topic/health/palliative-care [Accessed].

Israels, T., R.C. Ribeiro, and E.M. Molyneux. 2010. Strategies to improve care for children with cancer in sub-Saharan Africa. *European Journal of Cancer* 46: 1960–1966.

Jimenez, G., W.S. Tan, A.K. Virk, C.K. Low, J. Car, and A.H.Y. Ho. 2018. Overview of systematic reviews of advance care planning: Summary of evidence and global lessons. *Journal of Pain and Symptom Management* 56 (436–459): e25.

Jonathan, S., K. Pfaff, L. Hamilton, E. Bull, M. Broadbent, and J. Echlin. 2018. Palliative care leadership in long-term care: Who are the leaders and what are their capabilities? *Journal of Pain and Symptom Management* 56: E29–E29.

Kaasa, S., J.H. Loge, M. Aapro, T. Albreht, R. Anderson, E. Bruera, C. Brunelli, A. Caraceni, A. Cervantes, D.C. Currow, L. Deliens, M. Fallon, X. Gómez-Batiste, K.S. Grotmol, B. Hannon, D.F. Haugen, I.J. Higginson, M.J. Hjermstad, D. Hui, K. Jordan, G.P. Kurita, P.J. Larkin, G. Miccinesi, F. Nauck, R. Pribakovic, G. Rodin, P. Sjøgren, P. Stone, C. Zimmermann, and T. Lundeby. 2018. Integration of oncology and palliative care: A lancet oncology commission. *The Lancet Oncology* 19: e588–e653.

Kaasalainen, S., T. Sussman, G. Thopson, P. Hunter, S. Sinclair, L. Venturato, L. Mccleary, P. Strachan, J. You, V. Bourgeois-Guerin, R. Bonifas, and D. Parker. 2018. Implementing a palliative approach in long-term care: A program evaluation. *Journal of Pain and Symptom Management* 56: E29–E30.

Kato, K., and H. Fukuda. 2017. Comparative economic evaluation of home-based and hospital-based palliative care for terminal cancer patients. *Geriatrics & Gerontology International* 17: 2247–2254.

Kingston, A., L. Robinson, H. Booth, M. Knapp, C. Jagger, and M.P. For The. 2018. Projections of multi-morbidity in the older population in England to 2035: Estimates from the population ageing and care simulation (PACSim) model. *Age and Ageing* 47: 374–380.

Klop, H.T., A.J.E. DE Veer, S.I. VAN Dongen, A.L. Francke, J.A.C. Rietjens, and B.D. Onwuteakaphilipsen. 2018. Palliative care for homeless people: A systematic review of the concerns, care needs and preferences, and the barriers and facilitators for providing palliative care. *BMC Palliative Care* 17: 67.

Knaul, F.M., P.E. Farmer, E.L. Krakauer, L. DE Lima, A. Bhadelia, X. Jiang Kwete, H. Arreola-Ornelas, O. Gómez-Dantés, N.M. Rodriguez, G.A.O. Alleyne, S.R. Connor, D.J. Hunter, D. Lohman, L. Radbruch, M. Del Rocío Sáenz Madrigal, R. Atun, K.M. Foley, J. Frenk, D.T. Jamison, M.R. Rajagopal, F.M. Knaul, P.E. Farmer, H. Abu-Saad Huijer, G.A.O. Alleyne, R. Atun, A. Binagwaho, S.M. Bošnjak, D. Clark, J.F. Cleary, J.R. Cossío Díaz, L. De Lima, K.M. Foley, J. Frenk, C. Goh, P.J. Goldschmidt-Clermont, M. Gospodarowicz, L. Gwyther, I.J. Higginson, T. Hughes-Hallett, D.J. Hunter, D.T. Jamison, E.L. Krakauer, D. Lohman, E.B.K. Luyirika, M.E. Medina Mora, F.N. Mwangi-Powell, S. Nishtar, M.E. O'brien, L. Radbruch, M.R. Rajagopal, K.S. Reddy, M. Del Rocío Sáenz Madrigal, J.A. Salerno, A. Bhadelia, S. Allende, H. Arreola-Ornelas, N. Bhadelia, M. Calderon, S.R. Connor, V.Y. Fan, O. Gómez-Dantés, J. Jiménez, C.R. Ntizimira, P.E. Perez-Cruz, I.G. Salas-Herrera, D. Spence, M.R. Steedman, S. Verguet, J.D. Downing, B.D. Paudel, M. Elsner, J.A. Gillespie, K.J. Hofman, X. Jiang Kwete, Q.T. Khanh, K.A. Lorenz, O. Méndez Carniado, R. Nugent, N.M. Rodriguez, E.B. Wroe, and C. Zimmerman. 2018. Alleviating the access abyss in palliative care and pain relief–an imperative of universal health coverage: The Lancet commission report. *The Lancet* 391: 1391–1454.

Krakauer, E.L., T.P. Nguyen, S.A. Husain, T.H. Nguyen, D.E. Joranson, N.K. Luong, and M.A. Maurer. 2015. Toward safe accessibility of opioid pain medicines in Vietnam and other developing countries: A balanced policy method. *Journal of Pain and Symptom Management* 49: 916–922.

Krakauer, E.L., D.H.Q. Thinh, Q.T. Khanh, H.T.M. Huyen, T.D. Tuan, T.H.N. The, D.D. Cuong, T.V. Thuan, N.P. Yen, P. Van Anh, N.T.P. Cham, K.P. Doyle, N.T.H. Yen, and L.N. Khue. 2018. Palliative Care in Vietnam: Long-term partnerships yield increasing access. *Journal of Pain and Symptom Management* 55: S92–S95.

Kumar, S. 2013. Models of delivering palliative and end-of-life care in India. *Current Opinion in Supportive and Palliative Care* 7: 216–222.

Landers, S., E. Madigan, B. Leff, R.J. Rosati, B.A. Mccann, R. Hornbake, R. Macmillan, K. Jones, K. Bowles, D. Dowding, T. Lee, T. Moorhead, S. Rodriguez, and E. Breese. 2016. The future of home health care: A strategic framework for optimizing value. *Home Health Care Management & Practice* 28: 262–278.

Lex, K.M., P. Larkin, J. Osterbrink, and S. Lorenzl. 2018. A Pilgrim's journey—When Parkinson's disease comes to an end in nursing homes. *Frontiers in Neurology* 9: 1068.

Lim, R. 2008. Improving cancer pain management in Malaysia. *Oncology* 74 (Suppl 1): 24–34.

Lohman, D., and J.J. Amon. 2015. Evaluating a human rights-based advocacy approach to expanding access to pain medicines and palliative care: Global advocacy and case studies from India, Kenya, and Ukraine. *Health and Human Rights* 17: 149–165.

Luyirika, E., & S. Enarson. 2017. *One hundred and forty-five countries signed the 1951 Refugee Convention: Why do refugees have limited access to quality health care and end-of-life care?* [Online]. Available: https://eapcnet.wordpress.com/2017/06/20/one-hundred-and-fortyfive-countries-signed-the-1951-refugee-convention-why-do-refugees-have-limited-access-toquality-health-care-and-end-of-life-care/. Accessed 23 July 2019.

Macdonald, V., A. Verster, A. Seale, R. Baggaley, and A. Ball. 2019. Universal health coverage and key populations. *Current Opinion in HIV and AIDS* 14: 433–438.

Macpherson, C.C., N. Chiochankitmun, and M. Akpinar-Elci. 2014. Hospice and palliation in the English-speaking Caribbean. *Cambridge Quarterly of Healthcare Ethics* 23: 341–348.

Maetens, A., K. Beernaert, R. DE Schreye, K. Faes, K. Pardon, L. Annemans, L. Deliens, K. Hermans, and J. Cohen. 2018. Impact of palliative home care use on appropriateness of care and costs at the end of life: A Nationwide quasi-experimental retrospective Casecontrolled study. *Journal of Pain and Symptom Management* 56: e48.

Marti, I., U. Hostettler, and M. Richter. 2017. End of life in high-security prisons in Switzerland: Overlapping and blurring of "care" and "custody" as institutional logics. *Journal of Correctional Health Care* 23: 32–42.

Mathers, C.D., and D. Loncar. 2006. Projections of global mortality and burden of disease from 2002 to 2030. *PLoS Medicine* 3: e442.

Maurer, M.A., A.M. Gilson, S.A. Husain, and J.F. Cleary. 2013. Examining influences on the availability of and access to opioids for pain management and palliative care. *Journal of Pain & Palliative Care Pharmacotherapy* 27: 255–260.

Mcdonald, M. 2017. *Palliative health care in Jordan for Syrian Refugees – An HHE report* [Online]. Available: https://humanitarianhealthethics.net/2017/05/24/palliative-health-care-injordan-for-syrian-refugees-an-hhe-report/. Accessed 23 July 2019.

Mogul, A.S., D.M. Cline, J. Gabbard, and C. Bryant. 2019. Missed opportunities: Integrating palliative care into the emergency Department for Older Adults Presenting as level I triage priority from long-term care facilities. *Journal of Emergency Medicine* 56: 145–152.

Murray, S.A., A. Firth, N. Schneider, B. Van Den Eynden, X. Gomez-Batiste, T. Brogaard, T. Villanueva, J. Abela, S. Eychmuller, G. Mitchell, J. Downing, L. Sallnow, E. Van Rijswijk, A. Barnard, M. Lynch, F. Fogen, and S. Moine. 2015. Promoting palliative care in the

community: Production of the primary palliative care toolkit by the European Association of Palliative Care Taskforce in primary palliative care. *Palliative Medicine* 29: 101–111.
Ntizimira, C.R., J.L. Nkurikiyimfura, O. Mukeshimana, S. Ngizwenayo, D. Mukasahaha, and C. Clancy. 2014. Palliative care in Africa: a global challenge. *Ecancermedicalscience* 8: 493.
Paal, P., C. Brandstötter, S. Lorenzl, P. Larkin, and F. Elsner. 2019. Postgraduate palliative care education for all healthcare providers in Europe: Results from an EAPC survey. *Palliative & Supportive Care* 17 (5): 495–506. https://doi.org/10.1017/S1478951518000986.
Payne, S., K. Froggatt, J. Hockley, D.C. Moore, and L. Van Den Block. 2018. Advancing palliative care in long term care facilities (LTCFs) in Europe within the PACE project: An innovative educational and development intervention. *Journal of Pain and Symptom Management* 56: E70–E71.
Poort, H., M.E.W.J. Peters, M.F.M. Gielissen, C.A.H.H.V.M. Verhagen, G. Bleijenberg, W.T.A. Van Der Graaf, A.J. Wearden, and H. Knoop. 2016. Fatigue in advanced cancer patients: Congruence between patients and their informal caregivers about Patients' fatigue severity during cancer treatment with palliative intent and predictors of agreement. *Journal of Pain and Symptom Management* 52: 336–344.
Porter, R. 1999. *The greatest benefit to the mankind: A medical history of humanity from antiquity to the present*. Los Angeles: Fontana Press.
Pot, A.M., R. VAN Dyck, C. Jonker, and D.J.H. Deeg. 1996. Verbal and physical aggression against demented elderly by informal caregivers in the Netherlands. *Social Psychiatry and Psychiatric Epidemiology* 31: 156–162.
Powell, R.A., R.M. Kaye, H. Ddungu, and F. Mwangi-Powell. 2010. Advancing drug availability-experiences from Africa. *Journal of Pain and Symptom Management* 40: 9–12.
Powell, R.A., F.N. Mwangi-Powell, L. Radbruch, G. Yamey, E.L. Krakauer, D. Spence, Z. Ali, S. Baxter, L. DE Lima, A. Xhixha, M.R. Rajagopal, and F. Knaul. 2015. Putting palliative care on the global health agenda. *The Lancet Oncology* 16: 131–133.
PRB. 2018. *World Population Data: The World Population Is Growing Older* [Online]. Available: http://www.worldpopdata.org/ [Accessed].
Radbruch, L., S. Payne, L. DE Lima, and D. Lohmann. 2013. The Lisbon challenge: Acknowledging palliative care as a human right. *Journal of Palliative Medicine* 16: 301–304.
Radbruch, L., L. De Lima, F. Knaul, R. Wenk, Z. Ali, S. Bhatnaghar, C. Blanchard, E. Bruera, R. Buitrago, C. Burla, M. Callaway, E.C. Munyoro, C. Centeno, J. Cleary, S. Connor, O. Davaasuren, J. Downing, K. Foley, C. Goh, W. Gomez-Garcia, R. Harding, Q.T. Khan, P. Larkin, M. Leng, E. Luyirika, J. Marston, S. Moine, H. Osman, K. Pettus, C. Puchalski, M.R. Rajagopal, D. Spence, O. Spruijt, C. Venkateswaran, B. Wee, R. Woodruff, J. Yong, and T. Pastrana. 2020. Redefining palliative care-a new consensus-based definition. *Journal of Pain and Symptom Management* 60 (4): 754–764. https://doi.org/10.1016/j.jpainsymman.2020.04.027. Epub 2020 May 6. PMID: 32387576; PMCID: PMC8096724.
Reville, B., and A.M. Foxwell. 2014. The global state of palliative care-progress and challenges in cancer care. *Annals of Palliative Medicine* 3: 129–138.
Robinson, J., M. Gott, C. Gardiner, and C. Ingleton. 2016. The 'problematisation' of palliative care in hospital: An exploratory review of international palliative care policy in five countries. *BMC Palliative Care* 15: 64.
Roider-Schur, S., T. Rumpold, K. Kirchheiner, E.K. Masel, R. Nemecek, M. Amering, H. Watzke, and B. Schrank. 2019. Migrate your mind: The role of palliative care in transcultural cancer treatment. *Wiener Klinische Wochenschrift* 131: 191–199.
Scott, J.F. 1994. More money for palliative care? The economics of denial. *Journal of Palliative Care* 10: 35–38.
Sepúlveda, C., A. Marlin, T. Yoshida, and A. Ullrich. 2002. Palliative care: The World Health Organization's global perspective. *Journal of Pain and Symptom Management* 24 (2): 91–96. https://doi.org/10.1016/s0885-3924(02)00440-2.

Sercu, M., I. Beyens, M. Cosyns, F. Mertens, M. Deveugele, and P. Pype. 2018. Rethinking Endof-life care and palliative care: Learning from the illness trajectories and lived experiences of terminally ill patients and their family carers. *Qualitative Health Research* 28: 2220–2238.

Seymour, J. 2011. Changing times: Preparing to meet palliative needs in the 21st century. *British Journal of Community Nursing* 16: 18.

Sharkey, L., B. Loring, M. Cowan, L. Riley, and E.L. Krakauer. 2018. National palliative care capacities around the world: Results from the World Health Organization Noncommunicable Disease Country Capacity Survey. *Palliative Medicine* 32: 106–113.

Sleeman, K.E., M. De Brito, S. Etkind, K. Nkhoma, P. Guo, I.J. Higginson, B. Gomes, and R. Harding. 2019. The escalating global burden of serious health-related suffering: Projections to 2060 by world regions, age groups, and health conditions. *The Lancet Global Health* 7: e883–e892.

Smets, T., B.B.D. Onwuteaka-Philipsen, R. Miranda, L. Pivodic, M. Tanghe, H. Van Hout, R.H.R.W. Pasman, M. Oosterveld-Vlug, R. Piers, N. Van Den Noortgate, A.B. Wichmann, Y. Engels, M. Vernooij-Dassen, J. Hockley, K. Froggatt, S. Payne, K. Szczerbinska, M. Kylanen, S. Leppaaho, I. Baranska, G. Gambassi, S. Pautex, C. Bassal, L. Deliens, L. Van Den Block, and P.T. Grp. 2018. Integrating palliative care in long-term care facilities across Europe (PACE): Protocol of a cluster randomized controlled trial of the 'PACE steps to success' intervention in seven countries. *BMC Palliative Care* 17: art 47.

Strachan, P., M. Bui, P. Durepos, T. Sussman, and S. Kaasalainen. 2016. Starting the conversation about palliative care for heart failure in long term care: Development of a HFspecific advance care planning resource. *European Journal of Cardiovascular Nursing* 15: S57–S58.

Sussman, T., S. Kaasalainen, S. Mintzberg, S. Sinclair, L. Young, J. Ploeg, V. Bourgeoisguerin, G. Thompson, L. Venturato, M. Earl, P. Strachan, J.J. You, R. Bonifas, and M. Mckee. 2017. Broadening end-of-life comfort to improve palliative care practices in long term care. *Canadian Journal on Aging-Revue Canadienne Du Vieillissement* 36: 306317.

Turner, M., and M. Peacock. 2017. Palliative care in UK prisons: Practical and emotional challenges for staff and fellow prisoners. *Journal of Correctional Health Care* 23: 56–65.

Uceda-Torres, M.E., J.N. Rodriguez-Rodriguez, F. Alvarado-Gomez, J.L. Sanchez-Ramos, and P. Mcgrath. 2016. Informal caregivers of palliative oncohematologic patients: The invisible guests: An exhaustive review of the literature available. *American Journal of Hospice & Palliative Medicine* 33: 691–702.

Unicef, W. 2018. *Astana declaration*. Astana, Kazakhstan.

Vanderpool, H.Y. 2015. *Palliative care: The 400-year quest for a good death*. North Carolina: McFahrland & Company, Inc, Publishers.

Weck, C.E., K.M. Lex, and S. Lorenzl. 2019. Telemedicine in palliative care: Implementation of new technologies to overcome structural challenges in the Care of Neurological Patients. *Frontiers in Neurology* 10: 510.

World Health Organization (WHO). 1998. *Cancer pain relief and palliative care in children*. World Health Organization. https://apps.who.int/iris/handle/10665/42001.

———. 2014. Strengthening of palliative care as a component of integrated treatment throughout the life course. *Journal of Pain & Palliative Care Pharmacotherapy* 28: 130–134.

———. 2018. *Ten facts on palliative care*. WHO.

Wilson, R., N. Hepgul, R.A. Saha, I.J. Higginson, and W. Gao. 2019. Symptom dimensions in people affected by long-term neurological conditions: A factor analysis of a patient-centred palliative care outcome symptom scale. *Scientific Reports* 9: 4972.

Chapter 5
What Makes a Good Death? Acknowledging the Global Cultural and Social Issues

Pierre Mallia

Abstract We often hear about the medicalization of death; many people die in hospital surrounded by a clinical environment and interventions. On the other hand, there are countries where even basic morphine may be difficult to be found. Again, some countries have hospices, which are a luxury when compared to developing countries. Qualify end of life care should be seen as a public health issue on the one hand and a health systems problem on the other. They argue that it is a global health problem because 85% of the 56 million deaths worldwide that occur annually are in developing countries. It is a public health problem because of the number of people it affects, including relatives' wellbeing indirectly, and the large-scale population-based nature of some possible interventions. Defining quality end of life care is important, as the parameters used will need to be measured. There are common problems to end of life but they differ within the context in which they interplay with one another. A bottom-up approach is noted and proposed to help in the formulation of the cultural approach to end of life care. Such a contextual application will be more amenable to define what we mean by a 'good' death, how to implement care planning, how one can shift from cure to palliative care, and how truth can be handled in an approach to global end-of-life care. Moreover, the difference between what we mean by public health as opposed to health-of-the-public, end of life being more of a health-of-the-public as individuals rather than having a risk to confuse it with other terms such as community health, chronic disease, health promotion.

Keywords Good death · Quality end of life · Global · Public health · Health-of-the-public · Global bioethics

We often hear about the medicalization of death; many people die in hospital surrounded by a clinical environment and interventions. On the other hand, there are countries where even basic morphine may be difficult to be found. Again, some

P. Mallia (✉)
Medical School, University of Malta, Msida, Malta
e-mail: pierre.mallia@um.edu.mt

P. Mallia et al. (eds.), *Challenges to the Global Issue of End of Life Care*, Advancing Global Bioethics 17, https://doi.org/10.1007/978-3-030-86386-9_5

countries have hospices, which are a luxury when compared to the developing world. Many books are written about the concern the west has about the quality and hospitalisation of death (Gawande 2015a, Warraich 2017, Nutik Zitter 2017, O'Mahony 2016). The World Health Organisation has seen quality end of life care as a global public health concern and a health systems problem (the latter being dealt with partially in Chap. 16). It is a global problem because 85% of the 56 million people dying worldwide annually are in developing countries and a public health concern because of the number of people it affects in terms of well-being (Singer and Bowman 2002). In this context it is difficult to assess what is a 'good' death from a cultural point of view. Certainly, understanding the epidemiology, cultures and the systems which countries are capable of or have the capacity for can help in directing the answer to what we mean by what the WHO has called a 'public health' issue (Gafaar et al. 2020; Ling Lee et al. 2011). If it is a public health issue is it simply to provide basic palliative care, or is it something more? This chapter attempts to address these issues by tackling how the west has absorbed death into a medical care which is causing concerns and how we can 'go back' to having a good death, but also looking at the different challenges faced by developing countries globally so as not to fall into the same trap. As we have seen, Singer and Bowman note that of the 56 million death occurring globally per year, 85% occur in developing countries. What is more important is recognising that the causes of death vary considerably between developed and developing countries with cardiovascular problems and caner being the more common in the former and infectious diseases (from HIV/AIDS, acute chest infections, malaria, measles and diarrhoeal diseases) in the latter. Moreover, these authors point out that most of the health care expenditure goes to curative efforts, with mostly urban hospitals taking more than 80%), whilst the majority of the population living in rural areas. They quote India as an example where an urban elite receive western-style palliative care which therefore reaches only a minority of people.

Harmonising end of life does not mean giving the same end of life care to everyone – just as bioethics has been said to have been 'westernised' (which is why we now attempt to move to a global understanding of bioethics. This is the same as reflecting upon equality as not being the same as 'sameness'; genders may be equal but still are not the same and (at least from a medical biopsychosocial point of view) may have different goals in health care to reach egalitarian ideals. Therefore, western people may speak about dying in hospital, in a hospice, or even at home and see how best they can have what they would consider a 'good death'. The very notion that we speak about a good death implies that death is not good as it stands even in the western world. In a way it has invaded, intentionally or inadvertently, hospitals that carry a burden which many who work there already perceive as not being natural or indeed dignified. This is perhaps what is meant by 'medicalization' of death. Conversely, developing countries may have lack of resources or good governance but the question is whether we ought to concern ourselves that they are given basic medical care only, or rather put questions on a level of where they stand now. It would be too simplistic to put the argument on palliative care only as what is usually perceived by this is medical/nursing attention, whereas palliative care not only includes other levels such as the spiritual but on a global level we need to speak about resources which are lacking and practices, such as dying at home, which can be improved without moving towards a medicalized situation as happened in the west. Therefore, harmonisation here means more 'harmony' in the sense of having a good death *for* that place and culture.

5.1 The Problem of Mortality

In April 2017 the weekly news magazine *The Economist* had an article on end of life entitled 'Mending mortality' (International Section 2017). Whilst we are speaking of the global public health problem of end of life, we are also concerned about how people die in developed countries. The article speaks about the many aspects of how death has changed over the twentieth century with lifespan increasing more over the past four generations than it has done over the previous 8000 - the average lifespan now being around age 71.8 when at the beginning of the century it was at 32 years. Many deaths were sudden or by infection when now death comes 'by stealth' and less than a fifth are sudden. This is the result of what the authors call the 'paradox' of modern medicine – where people live longer and yet doing so with more disease; death being rather a long process and often painful. Many people die in hospital often 'after pointless, aggressive treatment. Many die alone, confused and in pain'. Whilst they argue that the distress is unnecessary, they point out that 'reformers are overhauling how end-of-life care is delivered and improving communication between doctors and patients in order to try to bring about less pain and suffering with people having more control in planning ahead.

Whilst most death a hundred years ago used to occur at home, now the WHO estimates that it is less than a third that do so, with poorer people more likely to die in hospital. This contrasts with the 'egalitarian' way people used to die in the past (International Section 2017). This can be explained by how we take health care system for granted. Death is not seen as part of life as it was in the past and when it was shared with relatives. Now it has been taken over by health systems – people diagnosed with cancer, for example, are given treatment until one deteriorates and has to be admitted to hospital. Even with the increased awareness of this medicalization, it is the health care professionals who are trying to 'give back' the process of death to the people. The concept of Advanced Care Planning is a process developed by health care and not patients, with the intent of discussing with patients what their wishes are. It is health professionals themselves who are questioning the need for CPR and developing protocols to decide when this is not necessary. The British General Medical Council (GMC) guidelines on end-of-life, advises that death ought to be 'recognised' (General Medical Council 2010). One ought to recognise that a patient will probably die within a year and also when death is approaching within the week. This formal process allows better communication and care at the end of life rather than continuing with extraordinary, disproportionate and even futile treatment.

Patients, on the other hand, may continue to be in denial, hoping for miracle cures. With them, their relatives. It is ironic indeed that the diagnoses and management of cancer has moved so much forward but thinking about the cost (not so much as financial but emotional) to the patient being taken for granted. This was brought about by society itself as everyone fears death and hopes that something can be done. We do not discuss frankly which cancers have what percentage rate of cure and the average life expectancy, even in a world of having a 'right to know'. Our conception of 'hope' has turned into one where people expect everything that can be done to be done. There is a time for hope and there is a time for reckoning; a time for continuing to live as is feasible and a time to accept and prepare for that final moment.

In *Intelligent Kindness*, John Ballatt and Penelope Campling (2013) discuss how one can have improved outcomes with kindness not only at the end of life but in health care in general. They give an arrow of care going from kinship, kindness, attentiveness, attunement, trust, through therapeutic alliance and hence better outcomes (Ballatt and Campling 2013) p 44. This process reduces anxiety leading back to kinship - what the authors refer to as the virtuous circle. When speaking about the end of life they also recognise that most people die in hospital moreover they point out to recent report (NCEPOD 2008, 2009) which found that 'aggressive but unavailing cancer treatment was still being given to some patients too near to the end of their life', highlighting where 'healthcare professionals were judged not to have the skills required to care for patients nearing the end of their lives. This was particularly so in relation to a lack of the ability to identify patients approaching the end of life, inadequate implementation of end-of-life care, and poor communication with patients, relatives and other healthcare professionals.' The authors go on to state that society is particularly uncomfortable with the reality of death and that this makes it difficult for both healthcare staff and patients and their families. Doctors and nurses feel uncomfortable engaging in conversations about death and prefer to avoid it. Thus a task-oriented approach becomes more feasible.

It is indeed this last statement which has taken us away from having a 'good' death and indeed in understanding what a good death ought to be. By adopting more comfortable approaches medicine has focussed on disease processes and interventions rather than engaging in and with the pain and emotional difficulty of an approaching death. We have adopted phrases such as 'fighting a battle' – as if it were a battle at all when we all know that death is inevitable for every one of us. We therefore feel we have 'lost' this battle when in fact we have not lost anything but we can find meaning in death and even acceptance through this meaning when losing a loved one or even when our own death is approaching. Ought death to represent a failure or an accepted outcome of a normal and indeed good life. The fact is that death can be ugly and we do not know whether by all the interventions we have done to prolong (rightly so) the life of a person with cancer by a few year, whether pain, for example, is actually worse than it would have been had the person not been treated. Although we speak about the principles of proportionality between withholding or withdrawing treatment (Gordijn and Emmerich 2019) we do know that both health care professionals and relatives feel the emotional burden of stopping a life-support treatment more difficult than not starting it at all.

Hospice care has provided a welcome relief from this situation but it is certainly not sufficient even in countries like the UK, with Hospices being charities and therefore more common in affluent areas. The Liverpool Care Pathway, as described in another chapter of this book, was a well-intentioned NICE-guideline-approved palliative care pathway for hospitals to give those who cannot avail themselves of a hospice a better end of life care path. It failed because it was not implemented well and indeed the outcome entitled 'One Chance to Get it Right' (Leadership Alliance for the Care of Dying People 2014)is indeed meaningful as with any patient we have *only* one chance to give them a good death. Learning from these mistakes is an important process which helped us understand that end of life is not only important but can be and has to be meaningful in some way. It can be meaningful even to health professionals to know that they find meaning in their work helping people rather than having situations where, for example, doctors and nurses disagree on approaches and what treatment ought to be continued or not.

5.2 Global Bioethics

If one were to ask what is the point of speaking about and attempting to help resolve the question of dying in developing countries, when one is not satisfied with the way we die in developed countries, this would imply a pessimistic approach. Rather the fact we learned through our own mistakes of medicalization, can help developing countries not only not to waste time re-inventing the wheel, but also to cherish what they may still have in their countries which we have lost in developed countries – such as the possibility of dying comfortably at home. It is this 'dying comfortably' which poses the real challenge on a global level. This is not only because of lack of palliative care services but also due to lack of resources ranging from water supplies to medication as simply as pain relief.

There are various actors in global health governance ranging from the WHO to other UN organisations and NGOs, not to mention charitable institutions and churches. Other actors are actors and celebrities who promote causes. Ten Have (Ten Have 2016) (p 147) points out to the gaps in this global health governance:

1. Knowledge – there is no agreement on the nature of the problem.
2. Norms – there is no agreement on international norms and how to address the problem.
3. Policies – there is disagreement on the formulation, adoption and implementation of norms.
4. Institutions – there is absence of robust global institutions with sufficient resources and authority.
5. Compliance – there is limited monitoring and enforcement; no clarity about responsibility, authority and capacity to monitor commitments.

This is a cold shower indeed. He continues to point out that there are diverging normative perspectives, diverging policies and inadequate institutions. Global Governance Institutions have capacity [problems and responsibility problems. Having been the head of the bioethics unit at UNESCO and having started the Global Bioethics programme, Ten Have is in a good and authoritative position to pronounce these concerns. He is however optimistic; 'if one takes the dialectics of global and local levels seriously, much of globalisation is 'from below'. In this view everybody takes part in globalization. The 'global' is often constituted within the local. Globalization is therefore not only experienced passively but in many cases actively produced by groups of citizens, agencies and institutions at the local level. In this view, global bioethics does not merely refer to ethical values and principles that are transcending various cultures or are interacting with them from the outside, but global values are co-produced in interactions with the local value systems. The global ethical framework is, so to speak, also emanating from the fast growing manifold interconnections between people worldwide. Global values are 'post-universal'; they are articulated in the sphere of 'interculturality" ((Ten Have 2016) p 151).

Ten Have argues that this globalization from below implies a different approach to governance – it is rooted in local traditions and allows for the participation of many stakeholders, which, he says, includes also the vulnerable themselves and the excluded populations - Global governance must involve local people, a shift of power and resources from state agencies and global institutions to local communities. In many ways Ten Have is speaking about people power – how people can be helped to help themselves. This involves more actors, a broader vision of governance and different practices and leadership ((Ten Have 2016) pp. 152–154). This reflects the *reciprocity* and *fraternity* that many people strive for today. It does not mean that we leave them on their own, but rather is consistent with helping them help themselves as well. After all, humanity finds its meaningfulness in relationships.

Bioethics can contribute to health governance. This governance *through* bioethics involves four functions ((Ten Have 2016) p 163). These apply snuggly into the end of life debate. First there is *Regulation* – Bioethics is involved in the development of many guidelines, recommendations and declarations. Countries need to develop and adopt these regulatory frameworks if they want to be a global player in health. Secondly *Oversight* – globally a network of bioethics committees have developed. Some of these are highly developed; others less. But review systems, such as that of research ethics committees have become standardized and harmonised. Global summits of ethics committees exchange experiences. Thirdly Ten Have points to *Deliberation* – Governance requires that developments in health and indeed in science and technology, are discussed publicly. Dialogue and exchange of views are important, he asserts, as any development involves the citizen. Fourthly there is *Interaction* – Global bioethics requires interaction about values and ethical principles. Policies and guidelines apply to interaction between individuals, doctors with patients, researchers with research subjects, nurses with people in need of care.

He does lament that there is little follow-up and quality control about how they are applied in practice.

To these four, one can add a fifth – that of *Reflection*. We need to reflect on successful and of failed experiences (such as the Liverpool Care Pathway). Reflection brought an improvement in overlooking end of life care in the UK from the insight into the LCP saga (Saunders 2013). This can be shared with other countries which may be bound to repeat the same mistakes. The very fact of 'medicalization' of death is an experience with underdeveloped countries ought to be aware of as they may have less resources at their disposal. Ten Have does actually speak about the sharing of information, experiences and best practices ((Ten Have 2016) p 177). Reflection not only contributes to capacity building but also to how things can be adapted to one's circumstances.

5.3 Global Quality End of Life Care

Singer and Bowman have argued that qualify end of life care should be seen as a public health issue on the one hand and a health systems problem on the other (Singer and Bowman 2002). They argue that it is a global health problem because 85% of the 56 million deaths worldwide that occur annually are in developing countries. It is a public health problem because of the number of people it affects, including relatives' wellbeing indirectly, and the large scale population-based nature of some possible interventions. It is a health system problem, they continue because of the need for information on quality end of life care. They recommend recasting quality end-of-life care as a public health measure, to strengthen the capacity to deliver this (as a public health measure) and to develop improved strategies to acquire information about quality end-of-life care.

How we define quality end of life care is important, as the parameters used will need to be measured. It would be appropriate to put these down as questions, for example:

1. Where would patient wish to die (e.g. home, hospital, etc)?
2. Have medical and symptomatic needs been attended to?
3. Has an Advanced Care Plan been made and to what extent was it followed?
4. Have the spiritual needs been attended to?
5. What were the patients' perceptions of care?
   (a) Medical
   (b) psychosocial
6. What were the families' perceptions of care?
7. Has the cultural context been taken into consideration?
8. Has the cultural context influenced the management of care? etc.

Singer and Bowman make the compelling argument that it is a health system problem because we need to improve quality end of life care, but also an information problem because we need to assess outcomes – they had never seen information on quality end-of-life care on report cards. We need to be able to measure outcomes as part of the health system management.

However, speaking about end of life as a 'public health' issue can be misleading even to some health care professionals. Moreover, it gives the impression that we are emphasizing the medicalization of death. That this is not the case needs further explication. I have argued (Mallia 2015) that we ought to distinguish between public health and 'health of the public'. One is direct and the other indirect. Therefore, if I smoke a cigarette in public I am directly harming others. However, if I eat a hamburger in public I am not; at most I am affecting the public health budget. It is indirect. Whilst not going into the details of the argument it is worth pointing out that the distinction is important because for direct public health issues, such as vaccination, a utilitarian ethics is more appropriate. One can have obligatory vaccination. But if it is simply a measure of correct diet, then there is a limit on how much one can impinge or even penalise people who continue to eat. A more deontological approach is appropriate. This practice is recognised in public health but there has never been a theory which can distinguish between the two. The article was written in the context of disaster situations. No vaccination can lead to disasters in the sense of many deaths occurring which could have been prevented, and that it is therefore worth considering the minimal risk involved. Of course there needs to be parameters where and to what extent (e.g. of time) these ought to be implemented. In the argument of Singer and Bowman, the fact that the relatives are indirectly involved is a public health issue in the usual way we understand it. With this model it would be a health of the public issue. One can only offer services and not impose them. But in the case of quality end of life care, we have approached 'disaster' situations even in developed countries, with people dying in pain, not having a care plan, continued to be given active futile treatment to the end, and indeed not actively discussing and changing management from cure to care. In developing countries countries, many simply do not get basic medications, including pain relief. Invoking the utilitarian model of public health would be appropriate as it would make mandatory training of health professionals, even those already qualified, and mandatory expenditure on provisions – at least to the extent that dying is not seen as less important than the treatment of cancer, chronic diseases and emergency situations. It would also save on resources where dying people are given active treatment in emergency departments rather than recognising that a management plan has been set up and what they are seeking is relief from symptoms. It has to be understood that doctors are held to a standard of care and no documentation that when a dying patient is referred to hospital may only mean that they are seeking relief of symptoms, or simply a bed to die on comfortably with 24-hour care may lead physicians to the standard of care of treating them as normal admissions, with the added burden of tests, not to mention cost-benefit analysis.

Conversely the indirect effects of dying on those around the patient would be more appropriately a health-of-the-public issue. Help can and should be organised, and indeed the very formulation of public health measures such as planning ahead may help relatives in their participation in care and indeed in the bereavement process. Investing in the health-systems problem would be more appropriately a public health issue. Singer and Bowman point to the Boston-based Institute for Health Care Improvements, which focuses on the application of rapid-cycle change quality improvement strategies to the problems of end-of-life care. They rightly advocate that the next phase would be to focus on this public health issue at a global level. They illustrate how the International Association for Hospice and Palliative Care is helping developing countries build programs that adapt to local cultures and realities, and how the World Health Organisation argues strongly for the need to address quality end-of-life care and bring palliative care in as a public health measure. I argue that using the public health P/H vs Health-of-the-public (HoP) model would make this even more clear. The fact is that if we include all HoP measures under one title of public health, we would be diluting this authoritative nomenclature and in turn making it less convincing. One needs to perceive that giving palliative care is as important as a vaccination programme. This is even pertinent for carrying out research on end of life care. Zaman et al. note, in this regard, that a 'New Public Health' is that working *with* the public rather than initiatives *to* the community. It is important to distinguish these as the all-encompassing 'public health' title can confuse when we need to adopt a more directive and obligatory approach (e.g. to vaccination) than a more deontological one, working with understanding of communities, societies and values, rather than with biological models. A study in Northeast Thailand showed that biomedical theories of disease coexist or are supplanted by more traditional beliefs about illness and that family and community provide ample social care (Singer and Bowman 2002). In Latin America, in a WHO Cancer and Palliative Care program, physicians and health care workers worked closely with government officials which in turned created an exchange of knowledge and ideas about populations.

5.4 The Evolution and Future of Dying – Towards Global Good Death

The capacity for proper end-of-life care in developing countries must deal with poor administrative systems, extreme poverty of many patients, restricted opioid prescribing and minimal educational opportunities for health care staff (Singer and Bowman 2002). It should be pointed out however that these four problems are not only found in developing countries. Whilst there may not be extreme poverty in more developed countries, it is certainly the case that people from lower socio-economic classes may not receive the same quality of care. In the UK we have seen that hospices, being charities, are more likely to be placed in middle to higher class areas. To remedy this the government introduced the Liverpool Care Pathway, which in the books was used as an example of how a poorly managed through the administrative systems, and lack of training for health care staff led to its being misused. One was simply 'put' on the LCP without the provider seeing that it was a 'pathway' and not a check-list. There one may have had ANH and everything else simply stopped, which led to complaints that it became a Euthanasia pathway (Leadership Alliance for the Care of Dying People 2014, Saunders 2013).

The majority of spending goes to curative care rather than palliative care. Again, this is not only a developing country issue. Gawande (2015a, b) illustrated that when one measured outcomes, insurances were more ready to pay for palliative care services. The WHO (WHO 2000) showed that quality end-of-life care does not need a high tech approach.

What constitutes a 'good' death has to change on the emerging global palliative care narrative (Klugman 2017). It is generally recognised that what we mean by a good death is 'dying well' (Hayes et al. 2014). In the west this is becoming to include:

1. The place of death
2. Care planning
3. Care pathways
4. Tools to measure quality of care

This scheme has to take into consideration the cultural context where it is applied. The meaning of a good death, and therefore, dying well, may vary when planning care, place and any available pathways. If global end-of-life care is to become a public health issue however item 4, that of measurement, has to be a necessary tool. Less high-tech alternatives which developing countries have may prove not to be factors for dying well. Conversely one may find that in developed countries, concepts such as autonomy and choosing 'not to give-up' may be more evident. We cannot 'idealise' death simply from a bioethics point of view. When moving from bioethics to clinical ethics, it is like moving from pharmacology to clinical medicine. A pharmacist provides (some of) the tools with which medicine is practices. Even though a pharmacist may know more about the biochemistry and specifications of a drug, at the end of the date the doctors has to balance all that she obtains from the history, examination and investigation in order to decide whether to prescribe. Bioethics provides the moral framework – it can tell one whether they have a moral objection to a certain practice. Doing clinical ethics mean being non-judgmental and irrespective of one moral position handles the case in a similar way. For example, a doctor may have an objection of conscience to abortion but irrespective of whether one agrees or disagrees with abortion, there is an ethical clinical way on how to handle such a case which goes beyond morality (CSA REF). Indeed research in bioethics continues to assess these outcomes. A papers published through the EndCare Project (Gordijn and Emmerich 2019) has shown that notwithstanding the supposed moral equivalence of withholding or withdrawing treatment, these two ethicists have shown that more bioethical discussion is needed on the issue as it is recognised through clinical practice that withdrawing treatment is more burdensome on carers and relatives and cannot simply be treated clinically in the same way. This may even have an impact on the legal position of withdrawing treatment as opposed to withholding. There is an interplay therefore between theoretical bioethics and clinical ethics. The latter is not simply the application of moral norms.

When problems arise, one goes back to the drawing table of bioethics to discuss the issue based on the experience and measurements in the clinical setting. One cannot do clinical ethics without patients. It is the *practice* of clinical ethics which tells us when and whether to approach a patient with the truth and what paths to suggest to people.

Zaman et al. (2017) have suggested that notwithstanding that there are cultural differences when interpreting what one means by a good death. The concept of the ideal of dying with dignity, peacefulness, preparedness, awareness, adjustment and acceptance in palliative care shows that these all depends on the degree of secularisation, individualism and social context, giving a different variant of what countries in developing countries mean by a good death. The focus is not on autonomy and rights but more on family, community and influence of religious values and the place of death. They note that the 'global mapping levels of palliative care development shows wide variations with regard to the preparedness of health systems' The situation globally varies between family-based palliative care alone, to isolated clinics, to a more developed palliative care systems. But the latter is in only 22 of these developing countries (Ibdi.). The length of time it takes to die has also to be considered. In the west there is a higher value placed on autonomy but even within the west itself studies do show that people from different cultures have different concepts about 'truth telling' (Searight and Gafford 2005). Zamal et al., in their literature review find that end of life in Sub Saharan Africa shows that palliative care in mainly a home issue and provided informally by women, the elderly and children. In Ghana, an emphasis is on the burial process rather than the dying person and the funeral is public. Conversely in Bangladesh people define a good death as that one where loved ones are present. The authors argue that these countries have been put in the 'waiting room of history', by this meaning that post-colonial countries have remained behind in many aspects including health care and by trying to provide palliative end of life care globally risks treating these countries by western standards not acknowledging the social and cultural values. The 'waiting room', which the autors recognise as those countries not so much influenced by European Enlightenment remain in an aspiring mode for a future (that of Europe), 'yearning for recognition' and being self-deprecating.

It is important here to note that Zamal et al. warn against a homogenizing of end of life care in order to take these cultural and social factors into consideration. This constrasts with the EndCare Project term 'harmonisation', by which is meant not a development of a homogenous end of life care, but rather a homogenous *process* for looking for important socio-cultural factors, a biopsychosocial approach, which will in fact take into consideration the important values of a given society.

There are common problems to end of life but they differ within the context in which they interplay with one another. Using the bottom-up approach, as noted from Ten Have above, will help in the formulation of the cultural approach to end of life care. This contextual application will be more amenable to define what we mean by a 'good' death, how to implement care planning, how one can shift from cure to palliative care, and how truth can be handled. An approach to global end-of-life care has moreover to recognise what we mean by public health as opposed to health-of-the-public in order not to dilute the term 'public health' and confuse it with other terms such as community health, chronic disease, health promotion, etc., which are all too often confusing each other. True public health issues ought to be one that requires immediate and appropriate timely management. They require a stronger utilitarian imposition on government and a function health-systems approach.

We need to:

1. Define what we mean by a good death in different global contexts
2. Implement Advanced Care Planning which will respect the socio-cultural values
3. Recognising impending death and when to change from cure to care
4. Recognise End-of-life as a proper Public health issue
5. Recognise the global context of quality end of life care which include systems, information gathering, and cultural contexts
6. Stop medicalizing death and implement palliative care strategies through public helath measures recognising how peoples judge the values within the death process.
7. Recognise, hence, the bottom-up approach which bioethics has to offer.

References

Ballatt, J., and P. Campling. 2013. *Intelligent kindness. Reforming the culture of health care*. London: RCPsych Publications.

Gafaar, T.O., M. Perambili, O. Henke, J.R. Nickenig Vissoci, B.T. Mmbaga, and C. Staton. 2020. *Good death: an explanatory study on perceptions and attitudes of patients, relatives, and health care providers, in Northern Tanzania*. https://doi.org/10.1371/journal.pone.0233494.

Gawande, A. 2015a. *Being mortal. Illness, medicine, and what matters in the end*. London: Profile Books in association with Wellcome Collection.

———. 2015b. Quantity and quality of life. Duties of care in life-limiting illness. *Journal of the American Medical Association* 315 (3): 267–269.

General Medical Council. 2010. *Treatment and care towards the end of life. Good practice in decision making*. London: General Medical Council.

Gordijn, B., and N. Emmerich. 2019. Beyond the equivalent thesis: How to think about the ethics of withdrawing and withholding life-saving treatment. *Theoretical Medicine and Bioethics* 40 (1): 21–41.

Hayes, A., C. Henry, M. Holloway, K. Lindsey, E. Sherwin, and T. Smith. 2014. *Pathways through Care at the end of life. A guide to person-centred care*. London/Philadelphia: Jessica Kingsley Publishers.

International Section: End-of-Life "Mending Mortality", 2017, *The Economist*, April 29th issue.

Klugman, C. 2017. *End of life in global perspective*. http://www.bioethics.net/2017/05/end-of-life-n-global-perspective/

Leadership Alliance for the Care of Dying People. 2014. *One chance to get it right*. London: Gateway Publications.

Ling Lee, G., I. Mun Hong Woo, and C. Goh. 2011. Understanding the concept of a 'good death' among bereaved family caregivers of cancer patients in Singapore. *Palliative and Supportive Care* 11: 37–46.

Mallia, P. 2015. Towards an ethical theory in disaster situations. *Medicine, Health Care and Philosophy* 18: 3–11.

NCEPOD 2008, *Systemic anti-cancer therapy: For better, for worse? National enquiry into patient outcomes and deaths*. NCEPOD.
——— 2009, *Death in acute hospitals: Caring to the end? National confidential enquiry into patient outcomes and deaths*, UK.
Nutik Zitter, J. 2017. *Extreme measure. Finding a better path to the end of life*. New York: Avery.
O'Mahony, S. 2016. *The way we die now*. London: Head of Zeus Ltd.
Saunders, J. 2013. The Liverpool care pathway. *Journal of the Malta College of Family Doctors* 2 (2): 5-5-10.
Searight, H., and J. Gafford. 2005. Cultural diversity at the end of life: Issues and guidelines for family physicians. *American Family Physician* 71 (3): 515–522.
Singer, P.A., and K.W. Bowman. 2002. Quality ned-of-life care: A global perspective. *BMC Palliative Care* 1 (4).
Ten Have, H. 2016. *Global bioethics. An introduction*. London/New York: Routledge.
Warraich, H. 2017. *Modern death. How medicine changed the end of life*. London: Duckworth Overlook.
WHO. 2000. *World health report annex table 3*, 164–167. Geneva: World Health Organisation.
Zaman, S., H. Inbadas, A. Whitelaw, and D. Clark. 2017. Common or multiple futures for end of life care around the world? Ideas from 'waiting room of history'. *Social Science & Mediciine* 172: 72–79.

Part II
Professional Issues

Chapter 6
Medical Decision-Making at the End of Life

Andrew Thorns and Dominique Wakefield

Abstract In this chapter the authors describe the ethical challenges facing clinicians at the end of life with a particular view to global challenges. A principled approach is taken to objectively assess patients and their wishes, incorporating that of the family. Whilst looking at the global wider context, the authors focus also on the specific nature of tackling issues of respecting the autonomy of patients, the principles of beneficence and non-maleficence, and justice in health care with respect to end-of-life decisions. The moral challenges involved and withdrawing of treatment can be very culturally elusive but can have common ground when taking an approach appropriate to the context of patients and their families.

6.1 Objectives for the Chapter

In this chapter we shall describe the ethical challenges facing clinicians when working with patients approaching the end of their life and their families. Readers will be able to identify why some clinicians as well as patients and their families find this specific area of practice more challenging. This will enable readers to evaluate how they can overcome these difficulties and how patient care may improve as a result.

6.2 Structure of the Chapter

Ethical dilemmas are frequent approaching the end of life but mostly resolvable. This chapter will help clinicians to achieve this in a series of steps.

A. Thorns · D. Wakefield (✉)
Department of Palliative Care, Guy's and St Thomas' NHS Foundation Trust, London, UK

P. Mallia et al. (eds.), *Challenges to the Global Issue of End of Life Care*, Advancing Global Bioethics 17, https://doi.org/10.1007/978-3-030-86386-9_6

Firstly to understand the background as to why clinicians, patients and their families may struggle with decision making when approaching the end of life. It is essential that clinicians seek to understand the values and views influenced by lived experience, faith, local cultures and resources

Secondly to put them in a context of the wider challenges health care faces in their locality. The different challenges faced in well-resourced and poorly resourced areas will make a significant difference to approach

Thirdly to use a framework to clarify the dilemma and be clear on the question they are trying to answer

Fourthly, to have a good understanding of the professional guidance in the area in the area of practice

Finally to effectively communicate with those involved so that they feel their views and beliefs have been heard and have been taken into account with the result that often complicated situations are better understood.

We shall start by looking at healthcare in a wider context and the reasons for people's reactions and behaviours before moving onto the frameworks, guidance and communication.

6.3 Ethical Decision Making in a Global Context

Health care practice is increasingly being influenced by internationalisation (sharing of people and ideas across borders) and also globalisation (the spread of cultures) (Mallia 2018). The question we need to then ask ourselves is whether from this we can develop global ethics? A harmonisation of practice and theory is an enticing idea. However, the challenges of bringing together the religions of the world, the various legal systems, cultures, public perceptions and applying the same ethical approaches to all countries where resources vary so dramatically are great.

There are issues of language, power, gender, oppression, to name but a few. We need to consider: beliefs about illness, dying and death; folk and popular health care practices; language and cultural practices (rituals, ceremonies and spirituality); and social organisation (families, kin and community) (Fried 1999). All of which will vary over the world. People will be marginalised according the level of palliative care they will receive by imprisonment, geography or culture.

However, one area that we can unite on is the increasing challenge of population change and resource shortage.

The number of people dying is increasing and the number of people dying at older age in particular. The developed world is seeing an increase in people with multi-morbidities. This trend is starting to be seen across the globe (World Health Organisation 2011).

In the UK, for example, the number of deaths is predicted to rise by 25% by 2040, the majority of which are in the over 85 age group (Sleeman et al. 2018). This is a cause for concern for us all. Health planners need to decide how to use scarce resources and frontline clinicians need to decide how their practice needs to change to meet this need. As part of any aspirations to achieve a good quality of life up until death and not just a good death. Such aspirations are perhaps at odds with the institutional and professionalisation of death seen across Western societies. Where complex healthcare systems are liable to overpower the spiritual cultural and community aspects of personhood that are still maintained in resource poor areas of the world (Stjernsward and Clark 2004).

In low-income countries communicable diseases such as diarrhoeal diseases and malaria are more likely to cause death and often at an early age compared to higher-income countries. Whilst Ischaemic heart disease and stroke feature in the top five causes of death for most countries globally, the cost and/or geography will put many treatments for these non-communicable and communicable diseases out of reach in low-income countries (WHO 2020). The dilemmas in well-resourced systems over which treatment to pursue or when to stop invasive medical therapies may likely therefore apply with less frequency. Irrespective there will be distress for the patient, family and health care professional's involved when aware of the potential treatment and/or care options available were it not for cost or geographical limitations. The scope of the morals of fair distribution of resource globally is beyond the scope of this chapter but is something all should be working to improve upon.

There are also differences to be considered when contrasting universal healthcare coverage with direct payments, with acknowledgement that even those with some form of health insurance may need to contribute or 'top up' depending on their coverage (World Health Organisation 2010). Systems that require payments to be made by patients at moments of need are likely to generate additional pressures on both patients and healthcare professionals and may negatively impact on the doctor-patient relationship. The options to consult different healthcare providers, for second opinions or varying levels of expertise, will also be limited by geography and the healthcare infrastructure of where you live. With remote locations or limited funding meaning that in some places there may only be one accessible doctor in contrast to populated locations with a vast array of healthcare providers to select from based on a patient's preference, to include when seeking a doctor that supports a patients request for certain treatments or interventions that might have been declined elsewhere.

In terms of ethical decision making there are universal approaches that are helpful and we hope to share some of these in this chapter. However, these will be subject to individual interpretation and application so the "right answer" is likely to still vary according to local policy, law and culture.

It is not feasible to capture all the global variations in ethical and legal interpretations that can be applied to medical decision-making within the scope of this chapter. Instead, the focus will be on a more practical approach to ethics, identifying the differences between well-resourced and less well-resourced systems where applicable.

6.4 Our Reactions to the Thought of Death and How This Affects Decision Making

A place to start for clinicians is to look within; after all the one certainty in life is death. As Lieberman puts it "we all know we are going to die but just don't expect it to be in our life time".

The terror management theory of death initially proposed by Ernest Becker and later expanded by Soloman et al. (2015) centres around the hypothesis that we are built with an evolutionary fear of dying.

Solomon and colleagues (2015) also theorised how humans manage the fear of death. They postulate that we construct our own reality and meanings – our own cultures. Something we can share with others close to us. Something that gives value and meaning. In all cultures there is a theme of immortality whether this is in the next world or in the form of a legacy that can be left behind. Each society has developed its own set of rules of how to behave or what is expected.

Solomon and colleagues demonstrated the importance of their theory by identifying behaviour and attitudinal change in participants exposed to reminders of death, for example when questioned in front of funeral directors or cemeteries. When working with patients approaching the end of their lives we as health care professionals will need to be mindful of this on two accounts. First our own fears and the way the thought of death affects our own behaviours and attitudes. Secondly the corresponding effect this will have on those we are caring for.

We need to reflect upon our own fears as part of efforts to find meaningful ways in which to engage in discussion with patients and their families about death and dying. Appreciating also, the fears and coping mechanisms that patients and families may exhibit consciously or subconsciously.

As an example, The Royal College of Physicians in London interviewed senior doctors and identified a reluctance to discuss issues around death (Bailey and Cogle 2018). The report quite rightly calls for a change in practice.

It is important to acknowledge that each citizen on this planet will have individualised views on death and its meaning. Therefore there are no set economic, cultural or religious frameworks that can be applied to generalise such views. There is certainly variation in societies as to the experience of witnessing death, with those in higher-income countries more likely to die in hospital or care home settings as opposed to at home with, therefore, a greater likelihood of family and friends being present to witness and share in the dying phase. Whether seeing death more frequently throughout one's life alters ones perception or fear of death remains uncertain. But it is important to consider this as part of exploring the thoughts and possibly fears amongst our patients, recognising any experience in their lives is likely to inform their thoughts on death and dying.

And why is this so important in this chapter on ethics? We will see that early discussion and advance care planning can have significant benefits for patients and those important to them. A by-product of such discussions can also include use of health services more aligned to the patients preferences and values as opposed to use shaped by systems and protocols. Therefore, we have a moral obligation as clinicians to explore sensitivity what is important to patients in acknowledgement of their mortality directly or indirectly.

6.5 Designing Containers of Care That Best Help the Patient and Those Close to Them

How should we as professionals achieve meaningful discussions about death and planning for the future? I shall first look at a theoretical approach, as put forward by Michael Kearney (Kearney 2011), before examining the skills in ethical decision making and communication that will help to achieve this.

From a developed world perspective Kearney explores the reaction of the id, soul or spirit of a person when faced with death. The person's id sees death being the dark, frightening, unknown thing below which it is trying desperately keep away from. He proposes that a container of care, which is built around the fearful id, provides the support required for the id to be gradually lowered down into the darkness(see Fig. 6.1). The type of container can vary from person to person. Sometimes a close all-encompassing container meeting every need, sometimes a looser arrangement available in the background if needed.

A number of authors support this theoretical model describing the importance of the patients journey. For example Cicely Saunders described her ambition that patients should" live until you die" or Gawande (2017) "it is not about a good death but living until you die". Solomon interprets the ability of palliative care teams to keep value in life whilst not denying death as the "magic of palliative care" and he

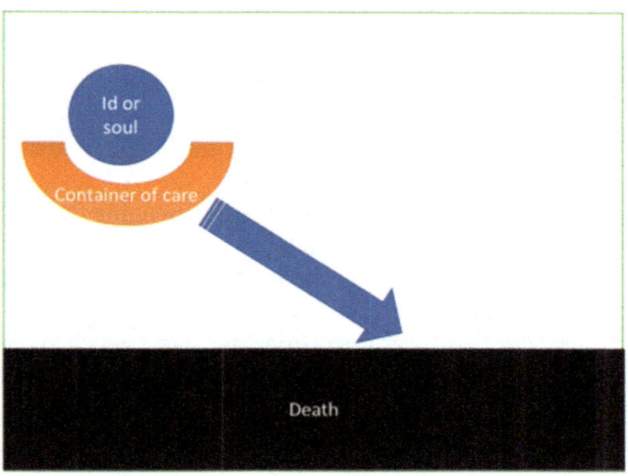

Diagram demonstrating how the container of care helps the journey of the id or soul to darkness of death

Fig. 6.1 A diagram demonstrating how the container or care helps the journey of the id, soul or spirit to the darkness of death

quotes Albert Camus in his Notebooks: "If you come to terms with death thereafter anything is possible" (Soloman et al. 2015) . Whilst there are no experimental studies the model is helpful in day to day practice.

This theoretical construct provides a basis on which to consider ones approach to supporting a dying person. We can see how a theoretical container of care may help achieve the goals that we seek and the road that patients and families need to tread but how are we going to do this practically?

This will require a range of skills and will encompass a number of chapters in this book, but, perhaps a fundamental to all is to ensure that the right decisions are being made in collaboration with what the patient would see as their overall benefit. The approach to how these decisions are made and communicated will be key to building a safe container around the person. If we don't approach these decisions with the knowledge and empathic skills to see through others' eyes, recognising what is important in their culture or belief systems on their journey, we are likely to fail.

6.6 The Moral Challenges We Face at the End of Life

The moral challenges we face at end of life include:

- Euthanasia and requests to end life
- Telling the truth
- Confidentiality
- Do Not Attempt Cardiopulmonary Resuscitation (DNACPR)
- Risk of shortening life with opioids and sedatives
- Clinically assisted hydration and nutrition at the end of life
- Capacity assessment
- Deprivation of liberty safeguards
- Withholding treatments - knowing when to stop
- Respecting choice
- Resource which could be financial, equipment, skills, medication or something as simple as time

These vary according to how frequently they occur and how challenging they are to resolve. Time and its just use as a resource, for example, must be the commonest dilemma we all face on a day to day basis though not limited to end of life. None of us live or work in an organisation where there is no limit on resource. Sometimes what might seem innocuous and straightforward decisions are made much more complicated by the circumstances surrounding that patient.

We need to be clear that the decision making is only part of the consideration. The communication and facilitation of any discussion is at least as important if not more so.

We shall look at common areas of concern using some case examples to base the discussion. We have not looked at the vital, wider question of how we best use our resources overall – which for the world is a key issue.

6.7 Withholding and Withdrawing Interventions

Case 1

Mr. A 52 year old man is admitted to hospital with severe chest pain from his advanced lung cancer.

While discussion about further treatment was taking place the patient's condition deteriorated.

The patient's views about Cardiopulmonary Resuscitation (CPR) were sought and he was in favour of resuscitation attempts being made, although this went against the advice of the clinical team who felt that the chances of success were 'negligible'.

The patient and his long-term partner felt it was a great burden to be asked to make this kind of decision.

Case 2

Mrs. T, unable to swallow following a stroke.

She has a feeding tube into her stomach but changes her mind and asks for it to be removed.

She has capacity for this decision and understands that by not having the feeding tube, to facilitate clinically assisted nutrition and hydration, that she will ultimately die as a result of its removal.

Case 3

Mr. R is 75 yrs. old and has had dementia for some years.

He is now immobile and unable to swallow.

A decision needs to be made about whether to feed him by clinically assisted means.

He is assessed to lack capacity for this decision (owing to his advanced dementia).

The above three cases provide some examples to consider when reflecting on how we make decisions when to withhold or withdraw interventions. If we consider the following framework we can see how it applies to each of these cases.

The layered approach:

- Layer 1. The framework or facts. What we are bound by
- Layer 2. The patient
- Layer 3. Formulate the ethical dilemma
- Layer 4. Establish the options
- Layer 5. Communicating and coordinating

Layer 1. The framework or facts. What we are bound by

- The law
- Professional Guidance
- Evidence base
- Resources available

Whilst legal interpretations and guidance may vary from country to country, there are likely to be key areas of agreement. For a clinician to work outside of their legal system or professional guidance would clearly be wrong. However, guidance is not always specific to every situation. We have already discussed that some treatment options may not be available in some areas of the world.

So, for example, in the UK the General Medical Council states

- "Doctors are not obliged to provide treatment solely because a patient or carer requests it, and should not continue with treatment that provides no overall benefit to a patient who lacks capacity to decide"
- "There is no absolute obligation to prolong life irrespective of the consequences for the patient, and irrespective of the patient's views" (General Medical Council 2010)

The clinician is then required to interpret this and apply to the situation they face.

All clinicians should work within the evidence base. It could be argued that we should all aim to contribute to the evidence base through research.

Layer 2. The patient.

- Their capacity for specific decision making
- Their beliefs and preferences
- Prognosis/outlook/likely changes in condition
- Other nominated decision makers where appropriate

It is unlikely that any health care system would go against the first point regarding a patient's capacity for the decision in hand. However, as we shall discuss the dilemma often comes when a patient is requesting an intervention that a clinician does not feel is in their overall benefit. It is generally accepted that a patient with capacity can refuse an intervention for any reason, to include when life is at risk, although such instances are liable to make many of those involved feeling uncomfortable as we shall see.

Capacity: a reminder

- Professionals need to assume a patient has capacity unless proven otherwise
- Capacity:
  - Can vary with time
  - Is decision specific
- Does the person have an impairment of, or a disturbance in the functioning of their mind or brain? If so…

- Does the impairment or disturbance mean that the person is unable to make the particular decision?

Mental capacity for a specific decision can only be confirmed if the person is able to do all of the following.

The person must be able to do at least one of the following:

- understand the information about the proposed intervention
- retain that information (even if only for a short period)
- use or weigh that information
- communicate the decision (by any means) (Mental Capacity Act 2005)

When a patient lacks capacity for a specific decision then local guidance and legal requirements will need to be consulted to see if written advance decisions or attorneys can be recognised and participate in decision making.

Layer 3. Formulate the ethical dilemma.

- Ensure the correct question(s) is being asked.
- Are we being influenced by our own perspective?

In complicated situations the dilemma often gets lost in emotion and tension. Effective team working with recourse to clinical ethicists should help identify exactly what the dilemma is and so what question needs to be answered. In less well-resourced systems or remote settings there may not be a team but taking sometime, even as a sole clinician, to reflect on what is causing the concern is to be encouraged.

Layer 4. Establish the options.

- What are the potential moral justifications?
- What are the practical solutions?
- What communication/negotiation/explanation is required?

The four principles approach developed by Beauchamp and Childress (Beauchamp & Childress 2008) provides a useful basis on which to look at the morality of a situation. Again, if available the use of an effective multi-disciplinary team and clinical ethicist will help to identify all practical and moral options.

Layer 5. Communicating and coordinating

- Communicating the options to those involved
- Coordinating and putting into action the decision making

Communication with all involved parties is often the most important and challenging part. The right course of action may be obvious to all but the heightened tensions and disagreements can be hard to overcome especially when discussing complex medical information.

If we now apply this to our cases.

Mr. A is a frail man has negligible chance of surviving a CPR attempt

- Would you support his wish to receive CPR in the event of cardiopulmonary arrest?
- What will happen to a dying patient if there is no valid record of a decision not to initiate CPR? Especially if they are going home to die?

The questions you would need to ask are:

Is a DNACPR decision justified and if so on what grounds?

There is an important distinction here between an intervention that is felt to be medically futile meaning it will not achieve its purpose, which largely sits within the clinical domain for decision making as opposed to decisions based on quality of life. It is generally accepted that clinicians cannot decide or take a view on a patient's quality of life – rightly this view can only be informed and directed by the patient themselves. We do, however, take into account quality of life when making larger scale decisions on resources – but that is a discussion outside the scope of this chapter.

What communication should take place and with who?

A landmark legal ruling in the UK (R (David Tracey) v (1) Cambridge University Hospitals NHS 2014) imposed a legal duty on Doctors to consult with and inform patients if their intention is to complete a DNACPR form. In addition to a duty to involve families/those close to patients in these decisions when a patient lacks the capacity to be involved. However this framework for decision making will not apply in all cultures or jurisdictions. Decisions about whether to attempt CPR at the end of life may not be as prevalent an issue in all areas of the world but serves as a useful example of how communication with patients should influence decision making. Perhaps, in absence of legal judgements or professional frameworks of practice, there may be a default to more paternalistic practice.

But in any culture patients should always have a right to opt out if they don't wish to participate in discussions that could cause emotional harm.

How would you approach a discussion with a patient and their family when you as a team have made the medical decision not to attempt CPR when that patient's heart stops?

Whilst outside the scope of this specific chapter it is always important to have ideas, useful phrases or explanations to hand.

So, if we assess that CPR attempts would be futile with no chance of success, what is the bottom line?

- Sensitive communication of the known facts about CPR will avoid most conflicts
- Discussion does not mean asking:
  - Is the aim to work together towards a decision?
  - Or towards clarifying a decision already made?
  - Avoid misleading people by creating an impression they have a choice when they do not
- A 2nd opinion will be vital if there is no agreement

For Mrs. T in case 2, this situation was effectively demonstrated by the case of Ms. B in the United Kingdom courts (Re B (Adult refusal of medical treatment) [2002] 2 FCR 1, 2002). Ms. B was being kept alive via ventilator (rather than via a feeding tube as per the example of Mrs. T) but had demonstrated her capacity to make the decision not to continue with this. The hospital and the team looking after her were not comfortable with this hence the case was taken to court.

The ruling was very clear that a patient can refuse any treatment for any reason provided they have sufficient capacity to make that decision. Mrs. T is therefore well within her rights. The challenge comes in being able to demonstrate the sufficient level of capacity in such cases, especially at times of heightened tension. This demonstrates the strong emphasis on respecting autonomy in the developed world, a dilemma perhaps less relatable for locations where resources are sparse.

The subject of clinically assisted nutrition and hydration, detailed in Mr. R's case(3), are common challenging dilemma's seen in practice. It is such a basic human need to eat and drink and one of the few things that families can support as part of their caring role. To see their loved one not fed or hydrated can raise significant emotion, especially when the person concerned lacks capacity to make decisions specific to this area.

Whilst guidance may vary from country to country, we turn again to the General Medical Council in the United Kingdom:

- "If a patient is in the end stage of a disease or condition, but you judge that their death is not expected within hours or days, you must provide clinically assisted nutrition or hydration if it would be of overall benefit to them…"
- "…taking into account the patient's beliefs and values, any previous request for nutrition or hydration by tube or drip and any other views they previously expressed about their care."
- "The patient's request must be given weight and, when the benefits, burdens and risks are finely balanced, will usually be the deciding factor." (General Medical Council 2010)

In this situation in the UK the decision maker will be the specialist in hospital and the primary care physician in the community. A decision needs to be made as to what is of most overall benefit to the patient. This should take into account all aspects of what is important to them not just based on clinical factors. Any advance care plans in existence may be helpful as we shall discuss later.

The right answer in this specific case is impossible to give in this chapter as it depends on so many factors, not least the skills of the multi-disciplinary team involved however two quotes may help to crystallise thoughts:

> "The benefits of a treatment that may prolong life, improve a patient's condition or manage their symptoms must be weighed against the burdens and risks for that patient, before you can reach a view about its overall benefit." (General Medical Council 2010).
>
> "The ethical situation is not that the patient is failing to drink and therefore will die, but that the patient is dying and therefore does not wish to drink" (Lennard-Jones 1999).

6.8 Comfort at the End of Life: Requests to End Life and Treatments that May Hasten Death

Mr. L has end stage heart failure. You don't expect an improvement in his condition. He is breathless from his pulmonary oedema and in pain from his immobility. He is struggling to take oral medications. He says to you: "you wouldn't treat a dog like this – can't you just give me an injection to end it all?"

The debates around assisted dying rage around the world with some countries legalising the practice in various forms. In those that haven't the discussions can be intense and heated. When patients use phrases such as this, clinicians are often on their guard and careful with their replies or even worse do not continue the discussion. However, if we were to put ourselves in the position of Mr. L would we not feel this way at least at times?

Globally we can agree that a pain free, in fact symptom-free, death should be available to everyone. To hear of someone becoming as desperate as Mr. L is clearly wrong.

What is it that Mr. L needs?

You can picture Mr. L, in a hospital bed, surrounded by things foreign to him, feeling out of control, fearful about the future, uncomfortable, suffering losses from the person he was and separated from those close to him. Or perhaps he is at home surrounded by a worried family in a village far from any health care? And if we put ourselves in this position what would we want?

Listening is the first step. The ability to ventilate our concerns can in itself be therapeutic. How often when faced with our own problems have we found by expressing them to someone else do we find we come to a better position?

With the application of a palliative care approach (not necessarily a specialist team) Mr. L's situation can then be improved. Removing some of his uncertainty. Returning to him some control. Improving his comfort. Working through his feelings. Agreeing achievable goals. Getting to his place of care and environment with support for the people close to him.

We are not saying this is the answer to all such requests. We know there are people whose desire for death is persistent and reasoned (Chochinov et al. 1995) but we must not miss the opportunity to listen as a first step.

If we continue to look at the case of Mr. L, following your discussion, Mr. L and his family accept he is dying soon and comfort is his main concern. You start some morphine and midazolam to control his symptoms. The nurse in charge is concerned in case these medications hastens his death.

We now must distinguish between interventions that bring about death and our concern for using medications that whilst helping relieve discomfort we fear may also shorten life. We need to be clear that appropriate symptom control is not the same as assisted dying.

There is no evidence that morphine or midazolam used in accordance with palliative care guidance shortens life (Maltoni 2012; Boland 2015). Of course, any medication used to excess or for the wrong reasons can result in harm or even death.

The key point is to use the medication in line with guidance (Association for Palliative Medicine 2012). If a clinician finds themselves in a position where they feel they may be shortening life then this is the trigger to discuss with palliative care services if they are available, as either there is a better approach that does not carry this risk or reassurance that what is being done is in line with accepted practice and so little or no risk of shortening life.

This area of ethical decision making is best summed up by the guidance of the Association for Palliative Medicine of Great Britain and Ireland:

Association for Palliative Medicine Position Statement.
APM position on the double effect (DE)

1. The Association for Palliative Medicine is an organisation of over 1000 specialist palliative care doctors working in hospices, hospitals and the community.
2. The Double Effect (sometimes called a rule, principle or doctrine) states that "The risk of a potential, known (foreseen), unintended consequence or side-effect of treatment is justified only if all the following criteria are met:
   - The intended effect is good in itself
   - The clinician's intention is solely to produce the good effect
   - The intervention is proportionate to the situation
   - The good effect is not achieved through the bad effect"
3. There is a misconception that morphine related drugs and sedative drugs bring about death more quickly and that doctors both know this and in some way condone their use with the double effect.
4. The APM refutes this claim: it knows of no credible research evidence to suggest that a patient's life is shortened either by opioids or sedatives when used in line with accepted palliative care practice
5. The APM believes that DE is unnecessary to justify the use or dosing regimes necessary to manage pain or distress in all but the most exceptional circumstances.
6. Professionals who are concerned they are shortening life by use of these medications should contact their local specialist palliative care services. (Association for Palliative Medicine 2009)

If there is no palliative care advice available the question to ask yourself is what is the worst thing that can happen? More often the risk of dying in distress and discomfort is greater than any risk of shortening life.

If we take a moment to consider those exceptional cases, then this is where we need to bring in the doctrine of double effect. If Mr. L is in significant distress with no reversible causes and with our only option to use medication that may shorten his life – what choice do we have? To leave him in great distress or take the risk that we may shorten his already short prognosis?

Intuitively, we hope all would agree, that his comfort is most important. Life, after all, for him is short either way but would go against our core human beliefs to leave him struggling.

The doctrine of double effect gives a moral justification for this position. It is supported widely but it is perhaps overestimated how often it needs to be applied.

We return once more to the importance of communication. The views of the nurse in charge (and all members of the team) are important. How this discussion is handled will be key to effective team working and hence best patient care.

6.9 Decision Making When Faced with Uncertainty

Mrs. D has Multiple Sclerosis (MS). She has been in a nursing home for 3 years and staff members there are finding it increasingly difficulty to manage her medical needs. She developed what the GP thinks is a urinary tract infection making her more acutely unwell. Mrs. D is somewhat confused and has very little awareness of her surroundings: she has been shown to lack capacity for some specific significant decisions. The manager of the home is considering asking for hospital admission to treat the acute problem however Mrs. D's daughter is resistant to this idea believing her mother to be near the end of her life and that she should not be moved. The primary care physician is aware of her recent general deterioration and considers that hospital is the better place to provide for the immediate care of her acute illness.

The dilemma of whether to move somebody with chronic ill health to hospital when faced with an acute illness is a common one and will be increasingly common as society ages and we are faced with increasing numbers of co-morbid conditions. If we push to one side the benefit an advance care plan would have provided for the time being, we can see from the perspective of the primary care physician, the care home staff and the daughter that all want the best for Mrs. D but how is the best to be defined and decided?

The professional staff are under an obligation to act in the overall benefit of Mrs. D. We have discussed already that this does not necessarily mean extending her life at all costs and would not require hospital admission if this did not contribute to her overall benefit.

Her daughter can help to inform the decision in deciding what her mother would have wanted if she were able to participate. Her views will be of particular importance as overall benefit is not just regarding Mrs. D's medical condition but all aspects of what is important to her.

A meeting to discuss and agree a next steps is required in absence of Mrs. D having capacity to be involved in decisions about her care or treatment in this instance. In the absence of a legally appointed advocate the doctor in charge is usually the decision maker and needs to ensure all relevant individuals have been consulted and their views given due weight. In England and Wales this approach is required under the Mental Capacity Act. (Mental Capacity Act 2005).

Professionals should be careful to not use their own perception of quality of life which can be tempting when faced with situations of great uncertainty. So how do we manage the uncertainty of these situations? What factors should we take into account?

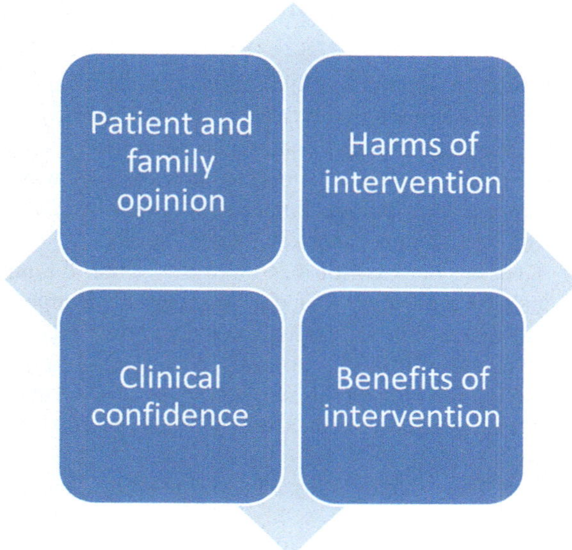

Fig. 6.2 The important factors to consider when decision-making at times of uncertainty

Uncertainty about the best decision to take is at the heart of these of these situations. Ethical models, research evidence, local and national guidance all play a part but at that moment the clinical team need to find an approach that will be practical and work for them. This has been the topic of much discussion amongst our local team and the factors we identified are illustrated in Fig. 6.2. Whilst similar to the four principles approach described by Beauchamp and Childress (2008), there are adaptations to fit with day to day clinical working.

In the respect for autonomy focussed developed world, patient (if they are able) and family opinion is key. As a clinician you will usually have an opinion about the future outlook with or without treatment and your confidence in this can be a key influencer. In some societies the clinician's view may be most important where a more paternalistic approach is accepted. Finally, to weigh up the potential harms or benefits of a situation can help to decide. A simple course of oral anti-biotics may be a reasonable intervention compared with extensive surgery with uncertain recovery for example.

The conclusion to Mrs. D's case was that all parties agreed that prior to the acute episode the prognosis for her was felt to be poor. The home manager arranged a meeting with the primary care physician and the patient's daughter. A decision is taken to care for Mrs. D at the home. Treatment for the presumed UTI is commenced. Mrs. D does not respond and slowly deteriorates over the next few days. She dies quite peacefully thereafter.

6.10 Futility and How to Apply in Clinical Care

It would be appropriate to expand upon the concept of futility here following on from the reference in the case of Mr. A (Page 73). Defined by the Oxford English Dictionary as "Useless, ineffectual, vain, frivolous" it does seem intuitive that at some point a potential intervention would not work and therefore should not be attempted. The dilemma comes as we described above, in how we define this point taking into account other key related factors.

Does an intervention become futile when the patient decides? Or the professional? Or does society need to put in limits? Dunphy in a thought provoking article suggests that with paternalism no longer being acceptable in Western healthcare that clinicians use futility as an alternative method to remain in control. As he puts it: "With the fall of paternalism, futility has become the battlefield by which the physician can recapture a measure of decision-making authority from the patient." (Dunphy 2000).

It is likely that in many less well-resourced systems rather than futility, it is the lack of resource which will be main limiting factor. Health care professionals frequently needing to decide how to distribute scarce resources in an equitable manner as possible.

6.11 Planning Ahead: Is Advance Care Planning the Answer?

We have described the human reluctance to discuss death and so to make plans for it. Yet we have seen in the cases how some earlier thought and decision making would have made finding the right answer easier, with greater confidence of being in line with the patient's wishes and less distress for others involved – in particular those close to the patient.

So where are we starting from with advance care planning? We have already outlined societies reluctance to talk openly about death and dying. Relatively few adults have discussed their own preferences to ensure their wishes are met. In the UK for example:

- 51% of those with a partner are unaware of their partner's wishes
- Only 36% of adults have written a will
- Only 29% have let someone know of funeral wishes
- Only 6% have written down wishes or preferences for future care (Dying Matters 2014)

It would be interesting to see if in society where death is not "hidden", as it has become in the developed world, whether the findings would be different.

Research suggests advance care plans can be effective. For example:

- Advance care plans (ACP) improve patient and family satisfaction and reduces care home admissions, stress, anxiety and depression in surviving relatives
- 10% of hospice patients with ACP died in hospital compared with 26% with no ACP
- Decrease use of life sustaining treatment
- Decrease hospital use and increase hospice use
- Increase compliance with patient's end of life wishes (Brinkman-Stoppelenburg et al. 2014)

Whilst not entirely proven, perhaps it should be argued there is sufficient evidence to say that as clinicians this should be an essential part of our role when working people approaching their end of their lives.

However, there are barriers. As Lund et al. (Lund, et al. 2015) put it:

- "This review demonstrates that doing more of the things that facilitate the delivery of advance care plans will not reduce the effects of those things that undermine them"
- "The findings underscore both the challenge and need to find ways to routinely incorporate ACPs in clinical settings where multiple and competing demands impact on practice. Interventions most likely to meet with success are those that make elements of Advance Care Planning workable within complex and time pressured clinical workflows"

Public campaigns such as those run by the UK group "Dying Matters" (Dying Matters n.d.) [image] can help.

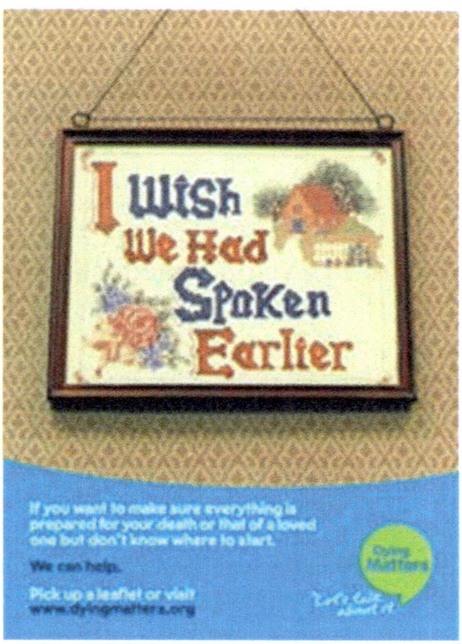
I Wish We Had Spoken Earlier
If you want to make sure everything is prepared for your death or that of a loved one but don't know where to start.
We can help.
Pick up a leaflet or visit www.dyingmatters.org
Dying Matters
Let's talk about it

Legal systems will vary as to how advance care plans can be put into place and enacted when the person loses capacity to make decisions for themselves. The type of plan may vary depending on the needs and attitude of the individual:

- A simple expression of preferences. Not legally binding but gives families and clinicians useful guidance for future decision making
- A written, legally formatted document stating interventions the person would not want. This would bind clinicians to follow this directive assuming it was set up correctly and there was no evidence that the person had changed their mind
- A legally appointed attorney who can give or withhold consent for interventions on their behalf in the event that the patient loses capacity

6.12 How to Have Important Discussions When There Is Disagreement or Uncertainty

Whilst this is not the main purpose of this chapter, as we have discussed this a key step in any ethical dilemmas, so worth sharing a couple of ideas.

- Research suggests that patients wait for clinicians to raise difficult discussions and clinicians wait for patients to raise. So we as clinicians need to take a lead.
- In an insightful study, Chiarchiaro and colleagues showed, that by talking about the person rather than the intervention agreement over difficult dilemmas is more easily reached. So, starting a discussion by "Tell me about your father" rather than "The chances of success of this operation is…" (Chiarchiaro et al. 2016).
- Listen for cues when talking to people as this is often the way people will introduce concerns for the future. A question linked to a cue is more likely to give significant information and we don't pick up on these cues the patient will stop giving them to us.

6.13 How to Grow and Develop Practice in End of Life Care

Ethical decision making does not stand still. Guidance changes, laws are developed and new evidence becomes available. So, in an effort to develop one's knowledge and skills in this area of practice we would suggest the following as areas for key focus:

- Keeping up to date with the evidence-based knowledge, law and official guidance
- Develop and practice skills to assess capacity effectively
- Working collaboratively within the team and involving others as required
- Communication skills to manage challenging ethical decisions
- Ensure emotional support for those involved
- Learn from each other. There is much that well resourced systems can learn from less well-resourced ones as well as the other way round

6.14 In Conclusion

We should strive for global harmonisation in good practice if not in the exact outcomes. To achieve this we need to consider where we are all starting from in order to make the most progress.

Your skills of empathy and communication are going to be as important as your ethical knowledge when faced with challenging situations.

We have focussed on the individual ethical dilemmas faced in day to day clinical practice. There are far bigger ethical dilemmas facing the world in terms of fair use of resources.

References

Association for Palliative Medicine. 2009. *Association for palliative medicine position statement on double effect.* [Online] Available at: https://apmonline.org/wp-content/uploads/2018/03/Double_Effect_0902.pdf. Accessed 19 Mar 2019.

———. 2012. *APM position on using sedating medication at the end of life.* Association for Palliative Medicine.

Bailey, S., and K. Cogle. 2018. *Talking about dying: How to begin honest conversations about what lies ahead.* London: Royal College of Physicians.

Beauchamp, T., and J. Childress. 2008. *Principles of biomedical ethics.* 6th ed. Oxford: Oxford University Press.

Boland, J. 2015. Is regular systemic opioid analgesia associated with a shorter survival in adult patients with cancer? A systematic literature review. *Pain* 156 (11): 2152–2163.

Brinkman-Stoppelenburg, A., J. Rietjens, and A. van der Heide. 2014. The effects of advance care planning on end of life care: A systematic review. *Palliative Medicine* 28 (8): 1000–1025.

Chiarchiaro, J., et al. 2016. Conflict management strategies in the ICU differ between palliative care specialists and intensivists. *Critical Care Medicine* 44 (5): 934–942.

Chochinov, H., et al. 1995. Desire for death in the terminally ill. *The American Journal of Psychiatry* 152 (8): 1185–1191.

Dunphy, K. 2000. Futilitarianism: Knowing how much is enough in end of life health care. *Palliative Medicine* 14: 313–322.

Dying Matters. 2014. *Millions leaving it too late to discuss dying wishes.* London: Dying Matters.

———. n.d. [Online] Available at: https://shop.hospiceuk.org/products/pack-of-5-posters-i-wish-we-had-spoken-earliert. Accessed 18 Mar 2019.

Fried, O. 1999. Many ways of caring: Reaching out to aboriginal palliative care clients in Central Australia. *Progress in Palliative Care* 7 (3): 116–119.

Gawande, A. 2017. *Being mortal. Medicine and what matters in the end.* New York: Picador.

General Medical Council. 2010. *Treatment and towards the end of life: Good practice in decision making.* London: General Medical Council.

Kearney, M. 2011. *The philosophy of palliative care.* Lisbon: European Association for Palliative Care.

Lennard-Jones, J. 1999. Giving or withholding fluid and nutrients: Ethical and legal aspects. *Journal of the Royal College of Physicians of London* 33: 39–45.

Lund, S., A. Richardson, and C. May. 2015. Barriers to advance care planning at the end of life: An explanatory systematic review of implementation studies. *PLoS One* 10 (2): e0116629.

Mallia, P. 2018. A practical comparison between Islamic and Christian end-of-life moral guidelines towards harmonization of end of life care. *European Journal of Bioethics* 9 (2): 185–202.

Maltoni, M. 2012. Palliative sedation in end of life care and survival: A systematic review. *Journal of Clinical Oncology* 30: 1378–1383.
Mental Capacity Act. 2005. *Mental capacity act*. London: Mental Capacity Act.
R (David Tracey) v (1) Cambridge University Hospitals NHS, 2014. London.
Re B (Adult refusal of medical treatment) [2002] 2 FCR 1, 2002. s.l.:s.n.
Sleeman, K.E., J. Leniz, I. Higginson, and K. Bristowe. 2018. *Cicely Saunders institute statement on palliative care and the Long term plan for the NHS*. London.
Soloman, S., J. Greenberg, and T. Pyszczynski. 2015. *The worm at the Core: On the role of death in life*. 1st ed. New York: Penguin Random House.
Stjernsward, J., and D. Clark. 2004. *Palliative medicine – A global perspective in Oxford textbook of palliative medicine*. 3rd ed. Oxford: Oxford Univerity Press.
WHO. 2020. *The top 10 causes of death*. World Health Organisation.
World Health Organisation. 2010. *Health systems financing: The path to universal coverage*. WHO.
———. 2011. *Global health and aging*. World Health Organisation.

Chapter 7
General Practice and Care at the End of Life: How Family Practice Changes According to Country

Pierre Mallia

Abstract General Practitioners/family doctors face end of life on a regular basis (Although they may sometimes be considered distinct, the terms Family Doctor (and Family Medicine) and General Practitioner (and General Practice) are commonly used interchangeably. Unless otherwise specified, this is the approach taken in this chapter). Whilst some people have arrangements to die at home and therefore require regular visits by the family doctor, others need the services of GPs to help from the very beginning when a diagnosis of a terminal illness is made. The chapter discusses the work of general practitioners and how they can help families and patients with services and indeed start the process of planning ahead. Post graduate curricula on the topic of end of life are discussed, especially for the case of the UK, and what is expected from a general practitioner. The challenges faced globally and suggestions on how they can be improved is also discussed within the context of home care and the competencies of general practitioners.

Keywords Dying at home · Core competencies · Satisfaction · Primary care management

7.1 Introduction

It is often said those who specialise in a particular medical discipline (such as cardiology or gastroenterology) know more and more about less and less, whilst General Practitioners (GPs) know more and more about more and more. This is particularly true when one considers the increasing range of knowledge that they have to deal with and the broad scope of this speciality in 'generalism' ranging as it does from child health to reproductive health to elderly populations. End of life care is one of the areas GPs need to be competent to provide, notwithstanding the fact

---

P. Mallia (✉)
Medical School, University of Malta, Msida, Malta
e-mail: pierre.mallia@um.edu.mt

P. Mallia et al. (eds.), *Challenges to the Global Issue of End of Life Care*, Advancing Global Bioethics 17, https://doi.org/10.1007/978-3-030-86386-9_7

that in many developed countries increasing numbers of people are dying in a professional care setting. Ballat and Campling (2013) (p 115) state that in the United Kingdom (UK) most people die do so in a hospital, and usually do so following a chronic illness. Ballat and Campling note that most people would prefer to die at home however, even though in the UK less than 20% do, with a similar proportion dying in care home and few dying in hospices. They quote medical psychoanalyst Anton Obholzer who suggests that the health service is in fact a 'keep-death-at-bay' service. Thus, even those who realise they are dying tend to attend hospital as their condition worsens.

The reason for the number of deaths taking place in hospital rather than in the home, is that:

> "modern affluent society is particularly uncomfortable with the reality of death, a discomfort that makes it a difficult area for both healthcare staff and patients and their families. Some doctors and nurses feel anxious about engaging in a conversation about death and prefer to avoid it. They adopt a more comfortable, task-centred approach, focussing on the disease process and the technicalities of intervention rather than risk emotional, interpersonal contact. At the same time, some patients and their families find it difficult to face the thought of imminent death and understandable want 'everything possible' to be done, reinforcing the pressure on staff to adopt aggressive treatment approaches, however minimal the possibility of 'cure'" (Ballat and Campling p. 117).

General practice is not confined to one body system or group of patients, although in some countries some do pursue a further specialization so as to provide for the needs of a particular group, such as elderly patients for example. But in general, GPs face most diseases at the primary care (primary contact) level. Whilst death at home was very common in the past, it cannot be said to be negligible today and there are increasing efforts to improve systems. One area of difficulty may be communicating the fact that not all that can be done in hospital can actually be attained at home. But once it is appropriately communicated that a lot that is actually done within hospitals may be futile or extraordinary, and may only serves to prolong a person's suffering, then the patient may be reassured by the availability of adequate treatment for a comfortable death at home. Thus, people will hopefully and probably opt to die at home, which has the advantages of one's surroundings and comforts with the added advantage of being close to friends and family.

GPs are specialist physicians trained in the principles of general practice. They are *personal doctors* primarily responsible for the provision of comprehensive and continuing care (Bradley 2006). They also provide care within the context of the family, meaning that they are aware of how the family affects the illness and how the illness affects the family. Therefore, besides promoting health, preventing disease and providing cure and care, they also offer palliation, which includes that which may be required towards the end of life. Moreover, GPs provide a biopsychosocial approach to health care which means that they can look after aspects which in hospital can at best be referred to other specialists within or without the hospital. GPs in the UK, according to one review, find caring for dying patients rewarding both for themselves and the families involved; they have good relations with community nurses but less satisfactory relationship with the hospital when patients die there (Field 1998). The core competencies of general practitioners are:

1. Primary care management
2. Person-centred care
3. Specific problem solving
4. Comprehensive approach
5. Community orientation
6. Holistic modelling

Whilst it is beyond the scope here to enter into detail of each one of these areas, they are almost self-explanatory. Furthermore, it can be seen that whilst these competencies were defined by the World Organisation of National Councils and Association of family doctors (WONCA), they can illuminate end of life homecare. According to Bradley the competent practitioner implements these tasks in three areas: clinical tasks, communication with patients, and management of the practice (Bradley 2006) (P. 4), giving a contextual, attitudinal and scientific research-based approach. The care provided by family doctors is, moreover, of a continuing type and it is often recommended that people ought to be able to 'name' their GP. The caveat however is that in some systems one can have GP practices where care may be provided by a group of doctors. In other systems, such as that found in Malta, one has a dual system – one of which is a true family practice service which is provided by private doctors (on a fee by consultation bases), whilst the other occurs through Health Centres where the doctors provide a walk-in service and also house calls. Whilst the latter is faithful to the core competencies, continuity may be provided through patient files and the patient does not always see the same doctor. In this respect it is argued that 'family practice' cannot be applied to this system of general practice. WONCA recognises the differences in many countries that GPs/FDs provide. Some may be more involved in public health or in tropical diseases, others provide some services which in more developed countries may be provided in hospitals. But the concept of primary care and the practice of community-based medicine based on GPs remains.

7.2 Core Competencies at End of Life

Although these are not clearly defined, we here identify them according to specific literature which are relevant on a global level. They can be listed as follows:

(a) Recognising patients who will die in the near future
(b) Communication
(c) Identifying and managing preparatory grief and depression
(d) Pain management
(e) Managing common symptoms
(f) Respecting preferences

(g) Making decisions with families

Recognising the imminence of death (be it within 1 year as defined by the General Medical Council Guidelines on End of Life, UK, and then recognising the imminence of the last few days). GPs can play an important role in timely recognition of death's imminence. A Dutch Sentinel Network of GPs studied how long before death do GPs recognise patients likely to die in the near future? Which patient, illness, and care-related characteristics are related to such recognition? How does recognising death in the near future, before the last week of life, relate to care during this period? (Abashi et al. 2011). Analyses showed that cancer and low functional status were positively associated with recognising death in the near future, and that this in turn was associated with fewer hospital visits, more GP contacts in the last week, more deaths in the preferred place, and more frequent GP-patient discussions about specific topics in the last 7 days of life.

Recognising that death will likely occur in the near future is vital for planning end-of-life care, decision making and allocation of resources. GPs did not identify that death was imminent in one-third of patients who did not die suddenly and it was completely missed in 20% of home deaths. Whilst the authors acknowledge that the dying phase will not always be discernible, these results point to the fact that GPs could use salient triggers in the process of recognition by, for example, assessing palliative care needs systematically.

Emery points out that more than 50% of those with terminal cancer wish to die at home surveys in the UK show that less than 20% do notwithstanding (Emery 2013). He asserts (albeit though a utilitarian analysis of cost) that it is worth studying what the obstacles are to allowing patients at the end of their life, to be cared for, and die at home. Dying at home, he points out, is associated with a 'good death' by many people. Emery identifies three main challenges – Identification of Patients, Improving Communication, and, Improving Training.

The Gold Standards Framework Prognostic Indicators (National Palliatvie and End of Life Care Partnership 2015; Mahmoud et al. 2008) have been developed to aid identification and it requires questions such as asking oneself whether one would be surprised if the patient had to die within the next few months, weeks, or days. This is followed by identifying cues in the patient. Once identified, communication with patients is essential especially when it comes to the preferred place of death. Improved training has been advocated and many studies show that doctors appreciate this training (Abela and Mallia 2016a, b). The chapter on Palliative Care in this book discusses this area more closely on a global level through studies carried out by the World Health Organisation.

Communication is essential not only to identify the wishes of the patient but also in discussing the advantages and disadvantages and the understanding on the part of the patients and/or family of the moral values of their culture/religion.

Patients need to understand:

1. What is the difference between home care and hospital care? In some countries hospitals may be far away and the care not optimal whilst in others dying patients going through a protocol of taking bloods daily, setting up of drips and other

measure which can verge on the extraordinary. This may be due to the fact that once in hospital people expect more.
2. The services, including the availability of the GP, which are accessible at home – such as hospice movements, local community organisations, etc.
3. The moral implications of these differences; the difference between ordinary and extraordinary care, the moral licitness of providing pain relief even if some perceive it may hasten death, and the legitimacy of these according to the cultural and religious values of the individual and the family
4. The feasibility of staying at home: is there someone at home with the patient at all times, even if to open the door for a community nurse? Etc.

Barclay and Arthur (2008) point out that the patient preferences in the UK for place of death are not stable. Longitudinal and qualitative studies reveal that the preference to remain at home can decline as the illness progresses and as the patient becomes less well they may opt for hospital care. It is unclear, they assert, whether this is due to the patient seeking better care, to save the relatives and friends the burden of them dying at home, or a combination of the two. Certainly the latter has become a cultural problem in Western families. Conversely, to be successful, palliative care has to include the patient's desire to remain at home, their attitude to death and dying, and the impact of the illness in terms of symptom management and the maintenance of personal dignity in the face of increasing weakness (Barclay and Arthur 2008).

7.3 The Global Challenge

In the 'Practice Guidelines' of the *American Family Physician* Smith (2001) lists a number of condition which ought to be present in providing palliative care and which can be used as a useful guide on a global level. Not all services may be available. Nonetheless one ought to guide oneself to know what can be offered and which are the areas needing improvement. The following is an adaptation/summary of the issues discussed by Smith:

What are the goals of Care?

Care should be coordinated across settings through regular communication during transitions or when needs change
Control of pain and symptoms, psychosocial distress, spiritual issues, practical needs
Preparing patients and families for the process of dying (taking cultural issues into consideration) with the exploration of available options.
Patients and families should receive ongoing information that enables their full understanding of the condition, and the pros and cons of treatment, plus that their values and goals should be elicited.

Care Team: Skills and Support

Members of the care team should be skilled in the care of the patient population to be served.
Effective communication skills

Effective coordination and continuity of care
Equal access to all patient populations under their jurisdiction
Knowledge of prognostication, signs and symptoms of imminent death, and the needs of the patient and family before and after death

Specialist-level Skills

Collectively the team should have specialist-level skills in the physical, social, psychological, spiritual, and legal aspects of medical care.
These include symptom control, management of social and practical needs, understanding comorbidities such as depression, anxiety, delirium, assessment of spiritual and existential issues, and ethical and legal factors of medical decision factors, such as the availability of Advanced Directives, and the more versatile Advanced Care Planning.

Support for the Team

The team needs education and training as well as care for the emotional impact.
Policies should guide recruitment, screening, training, work practices, and performance
Ongoing education, supervision, and support
Regular meetings for review and discussion of the providing palliative care in the community.

Support for the Family

The family should be educated about the process of palliative care and any respite services and be educated and assisted in providing the patient with safe, appropriate comfort measures and psychological support; they may also need backup resources.
Routine meetings with family members to assess understanding, wishes and address questions.

Referrals

Patients and families should be informed and offered other available services such as hospices, in-patient care, and community services.
Referral should be made to those services that meet identified social needs and access to care

Treatment

Treatment decisions should be made according to the goals of care, assessing risk and benefit and preferences of patient and family.
The goal of pain management is safe and timely reduction of pain and symptoms to an acceptable level.
Include pharmacological and non-pharmacological, and complementary therapies.
Barriers include addiction in long term care - managed appropriately by stepping up and stepping down accordingly.
Conversely carers should work with authorities to regulate controlled substances to ensure that drug abuse do not interfere with the care of patients who are in pain (such as the recent controversy over cannaboids which may be very useful to terminally ill patients who do not tolerate other medications such as morphine).

Care Setting

Safety
Flexible visits
In hospices a space of families to visit, rest, eat or prepare meals
Meeting with palliative care team
Privacy
Child care needs

End of Life

Availability of referrals for those who have not accessed hospice services
Recognition and communication
Addressing of concerns, hopes, fear, and expectations
Support for issues of life completion according to cultural and religious values
Pastoral care and its facilitation
Bereavement services

Ethical and Legal Aspects

The team and GP should be prepared to discuss and answer the complex ethical issues arising with persons with life-threatening illnesses, recognising cultural variations
Professional advice about wills and guardianship
Surrogate decision makers should be assisted with ethical and legal advice, such as honouring patient's wishes
Discuss dilemmas of withholding or withdrawing treatment. Although these are seen to be morally equivalent, people perceive them differently and ought to be addressed accordingly if necessary.

Smith also discusses Care Plans and Quality. Here they are discussed separately below due to their contemporary nature and significance.

7.4 Advanced Care Planning and the General Practitioner

Advanced Care Planning is a process of discussing with the patient, their care providers and often those close to them, the future care of the patient (Kite 2010). It provides a framework for the preferences of the patient. Because Advance Directives are not yet norm in many countries (and indeed having strict legal frameworks can complicate things at the end of life when decisions are wont to be reversed), end of life decisions for patients without medical decision capacity are made regularly with discussions between the patient's physician and the family (LANG, QUILL). Planning ahead for this eventuality is essential. Lang and Quill (2004) argue that the most common pitfalls in establishing plans of care for patients who lack capacity include failure to reach a shared appreciation of the patient's condition and prognosis, a failure to apply the principles of substituted judgement, and offering the choice between care and cure rather than life-prolonging treatment (which can often simply mean referring as an in-patient.

Patients, especially early on in the treatment plan, however, are often able to discuss planning ahead. Family physicians are in a position to integrate medical knowledge, individual values, and cultural influences into end-of-life care; they can best respect the capacity and autonomy of patients by allowing the patient and family to prospectively identify relevant health care preferences by sustaining an ongoing discussion and by abiding by these decisions (Crane and Wittink 2005).

Whilst the chapter in this book by John Paes goes into more detail on Advanced Care Planning, especially in the hospital setting, what applies in the hospital will also apply in the community. The aim of ACP is to fulfil the goals held by many patients, including,

- Participation in decisions about treatment preferences
- Preparation for death
- Achieving a sense of completion
- Being in familiar surroundings in the company of close family and friends. (Kite 2010)

Whilst hospital physicians have a vital role in identifying patients who have reached the last year of life (Kite 2010), communication and coordination with family physicians is important to achieving the goals intended by ACPs. It is important that both primary care and secondary care physicians understand, agree, and document Advanced Decision to Refuse Treatment (ADRT). This is not as easy as one can imagine it to be, but the role played by a GP who will not refer a patient unnecessarily to hospital when the time comes is not only essential but perhaps needs legislation back-up. It is important that primary and secondary care physicians work together to attain this goal both locally and on a global level, respecting human values and the right to be allowed to die without undue intervention. Such can be the case, for example, for a patient with motor neuron disease, who does not wish to live on a respirator, even if this prolongs her life by a few years. Moreover in many countries there is not the possibility of such treatment at home and the person may have to remain until the end in an intensive care unit, or at best in a ward. The GP has the role of finding things out for the patient and act as advocate for her and the family.

ACPs always act in accordance with the law but there are things which the law must clarify, even though they are technically lawful (or not unlawful). It avoids legal showdowns and reassures family and friends in the mourning process that no decision which verges on euthanasia in the mind of people, for example, has taken place. Protocols and published standards of care are important to satisfy that health care providers have not been negligent.

7.4.1 Patient Advocacy

Primary care physicians are numerous enough and strategically placed to identify areas which ned improvement. Both alone and together they can act, as the case may be, as patient advocates to improve protocols, standards, ethical documents and encourage legislations in this regard. The local Colleges and Associations of GPs can work with other Physician and health care professions' associations to effect change. A clear example is the case of the preceding paragraph where legislation or standards would be helpful when deciding about refusing life prolonging treatment and making the final decision not to refer to hospital when the time comes and be prepared for any sedation of distress.

7.4.2 Quality Framework

Countries ought to strive to have quality frameworks for proper end-of-life care and palliative care. Implementing pathways with due training and communication, for example, can give rise to distorted perceptions, as happened with the Liverpool Care Pathways. In point of fact, the lack of training and not following the 'path' may have made these perceptions right in some instances, as many British authors pointed out retrospectively.

Quality frameworks are important to link scholarship with action (Tan 2007). GPs strive to maintain continuity of care within an increasingly complex health care environment. GP recognise that they work and live in a highly complex world and not a purely mechanical one, and that the unique perspective and experiential knowledge that resides in ach family physicians in their individual setting provides the basis for therapeutic management at various levels. Of the health care environment (Tan 2007). Quality Improvement (QI) is a priority in health care. New research redefines best practice and health needs in particular populations, such as the elderly, changes (Booth and Snowdon 2007). Moreover, health needs in different countries change and this points towards important QI programme which needs to be adapted locally.

As principal coordinators of end of life care for people dying at home, such frameworks can highlight achievements and gaps (Booth and Snowdon 2007). In health care QI occurs through Vocational Training programme which lead to the specialist qualification of GPs, Fellowships of Colleges, Continuing Medical Education and Continuing Professional Development (such as taking a course in palliative care or communication skills) are the mainstay of QI in general practice.

However there are other stake holders in end-of-life care, including nurses, other health care professionals, patient groups, legislators, hospice movements etc. and last but not least the politicians who is entrusted with effecting change. Broad consultation is needed to improve quality of care. On the other hand one must assess the capacity of local General Practice services to handle end of life care. Capacity has to be assessed both at national level and on a personal (capacity) level – the GP self care (Snowdon et al. 2007). 'What is our capacity to provide end-of-life care at home?', for example, needs to be answered effectively for the system to work – acceding better to patient's wishes, and in the process allocating resources more effectively. The professions own uncertainty for the need for change can offer resistance (Flynn et al. 2007). A vision has to ensure, besides the capacity, the doctors are properly qualified and fit to practice, promote excellence and good practice, responds to concerns of the individual and works with the community and medical profession to identify and resolve problem areas (Flynn et al. 2007). The involvement of community ensure patient-centred responses, expectation of consumers, and health inequalities (Booth and Snowdon 2007).

Quality means that one has to focus on competence at all levels, from that of individual health professionals, to working as a team (Atkinson et al. 2007). They need clear and concise templates or pathways, training in these pathways, clear defining of the roles within the team, with regular face-to-face meetings and regular professional development.

In the UK, the 'Gold Standards Framework' for end of life care showed that its implementation enabled process of communication and that it was associated with a marked high quality palliative care in general practice, although there was a marked variation in how this worked in individual teams; but the general hierarchical doctor-nurse relationships persisted (Mahmoud et al. 2008).

7.4.3 Multidisciplinary Teams

GPs are an essential factor in a community multidisciplinary approach to end of life care, but one should not undermine the important role of other professionals with whom the patient and family also create relationship, without whom the GP cannot function effectively. Mahmoud Yousef et al. assert that multidisciplinary working in primary care is essential for delivering high quality end-of-life care in the community. Implementing can take time and in the UK the hierarchy remained. District nurses and GPs are shown to have different priorities and styles of multidisciplinary workings. Teams who have a relatively non-hierarchical working style rather than a rigidly hierarchical structure of decision making seem to be more effective. High performance practices displayed a clear shared purpose among staff for palliative care. Effective primary care therefor appears to require good team work. The Gold Standards Framework has helped in this regard when implanted, in providing the elements of the seven-Cs – communication, coordination of care, control of symptoms, continuity out of hours, continued learning, carer support, and care in the dying phase.

7.5 Knowledge and Skills Required of GPs at the End of Life

Acknowledging the contextuality of primary care and general practice, with special regard to end of life issues, considering the divergence of global issues ranging from lack of resources, distance from services, lack of clean water, etc., the Curriculum of the Royal College of General Practitioners (REF) is a good guide in this regard. It states that:

- An essential role of a GP is to help patients die with dignity, providing individualised care and minimising distress
- Many terminally ill patients prefer the option of a death at home
- Most patients die of non-cancer/co-morbidity in old age
- GPs must be able to identify patients in the last year(s) of life and their carers
- GPs must be able to assess patients holistically and compassionately and agree personalised plans for their future care

Team working, interagency working and communication are fundamental to good end-of-life care

Curriculum of the Royal College of General Practitioners, Chapter 3.09 End-of-Life Care.

Knowledge and skills guide (3.09 End-of-Life Care RCGP Curriculum: Professional and Clinical Modules 18 May 2015 p 183).

Core Competence: Fitness to practise

This concerns the development of professional values, behaviours and personal resilience and preparation for career-long development and revalidation. It includes having insight into when your own performance, conduct or health might put patients at risk, as well as taking action to protect patients.

This means that as a GP you should:

- *Read the GMC's document on end-of-life care with case examples*
- *Recognise that personal life events, such as deaths in the family, can make full clinical engagement a test of your professionalism*

Core Competence: Maintaining an ethical approach

This addresses the importance of practising ethically, with integrity and a respect for diversity.

This means that as a GP you should:

- *Be aware of your cultural values and/or religious beliefs which might make it difficult for you to be non-judgemental about your patients' decisions at the end of their life*

Core Competence: Communication and consultation

This is about communication with patients, the use of recognised consultation techniques, establishing patient partnership, managing challenging consultations, third-party consulting and the use of interpreters.

This means that as a GP you should:

- *Communicate effectively with the patient, their family and carer(s) regarding difficult information about disease progression and prognosis.*
- *Describe how to provide and manage 24-h continuity of care through various clinical systems*

Core Competence: Data gathering and interpretation

This is about interpreting the patient's narrative, clinical record and biographical data. It also concerns the use of investigations and examination findings, plus the adoption of a proficient approach to clinical examination and procedural skills.

This means that as a GP you should:

- *Describe palliative care emergencies and their appropriate management:*
- *use of emergency drugs*
- *major haemorrhage*
- *spinal cord compression*
- *anxiety/panic o dysphagia*
- *bone fractures*
- *hypercalcaemia*
- *superior vena cava obstruction*
  Core Competence: Making decisions

This is about having a conscious, structured approach to decision-making; within the consultation and in wider areas of practice.

This means that as a GP you should:

- *Apply best practice principles for end-of-life care in community settings, such as those described in the Gold Standards Framework*
- *Counsel and explain for patients, families and their carers:*
- *a holistic and personalised assessment of needs*
- *symptom control*
- *disease progression*
- *processes around death and dying*
- *advance care planning o normal and abnormal bereavement*
  Core Competence: Clinical management

This concerns the recognition and management of common medical conditions encountered in generalist medical care. It includes safe prescribing and medicines management approaches.

This means that as a GP you should:

- *Co-develop with the patient, carers and family an effective plan to manage the full range of their physical, psychological, socioeconomic, cultural and spiritual needs*
- *Manage distressing symptoms, e.g. nausea, pain, shortness of breath and confusion.*
- *Use appropriate drug/nutrition delivery systems, e.g. a syringe driver*
- *Prescribe effective drugs and suitable combinations of drugs, pre-empting likely side-effects*
- *Describe the conversion of drugs from oral dosage to other appropriate delivery systems*

  Core Competence: Managing medical complexity

This is about aspects of care beyond managing straightforward problems. It includes multiprofessional management of co-morbidity and poly-pharmacy, as well as uncertainty and risk. It also covers appropriate referral, planning and organising complex care, promoting recovery and rehabilitation.

This means that as a GP you should:

- *Summarise the principles of palliative care and end-of-life care and how these apply to cancer and non-cancer illnesses such as cardiovascular, neurological, respiratory and infectious diseases Core Competence: Working with colleagues and in teams*

This is about working effectively with other professionals to ensure good patient care. It includes sharing information with colleagues, effective service navigation, use of team skill mix, applying leadership, management and team-working skills in real-life practice, and demonstrating flexibility with regard to career development.

This means that as a GP you should:

- *Function as both leader and member of end-of-life teams, as required*
- *Work effectively with the community nursing and end-of-life care teams and teams from social care and voluntary sector organisations*

  Core Competence: Maintaining performance, learning and teaching

This area is about maintaining performance and effective CPD for oneself and others, self-directed adult learning, leading clinical care and service development, participating in commissioning, quality improvement and research activity.

This means that as a GP you should:

- *Understand the evidence base for care at the end of life, while also acknowledging that it is less rigorous because there are very few trials available.*
- *Understand the difficulty of running double-blinded randomised controlled trials in patients who are dying.*
  Core Competence: Organisational management and leadership

This is about the understanding of organisations and systems, the appropriate use of administration systems, effective record keeping and utilisation of IT for the benefit of patient care. It also includes structured care planning, using new technologies to access and deliver care and developing relevant business and financial management skills.

This means that as a GP you should:

- *Review the key national guidelines and policies that influence healthcare provision for end-of-life and palliative care, applying these compassionately to the personalised needs and wishes of patients, their families and carers*
  Core Competence: Practising holistically and promoting health

This is about the physical, psychological, socioeconomic and cultural dimensions of health. It includes considering feelings as well as thoughts, encouraging health improvement, preventative medicine, self-management and care planning with patients and carers.

This means that as a GP you should:

- *Identify and respond to the spiritual, socioeconomic and cultural needs of the patient, family and carers, in addition to their 'biomedical' physical and psychological needs*
- *Acknowledge the appropriate use of alternative therapies which individual patients may find provide comfort, while bearing in mind the evidence for their use*
- *Recognise normal and abnormal grieving, and its impact upon symptomatology, and provide support appropriately*
  Core Competence: Community orientation

This is about involvement in the health of the local population. It includes understanding the need to build community engagement and resilience, family and community-based interventions, as well as the global and multi-cultural aspects of delivering evidence-based, sustainable healthcare.

This means that as a GP you should:

- *Summarise the social benefits and services available to patients and carer(s)*
- *Describe the current population trends in the prevalence of terminal illness in the community*
- *Explain the importance of the social and psychological impact of terminal illness and dying on the patient's community, such as their wider family, friends, dependents, employers and work colleagues.*

References

Abashi, E., M. Echteld, L. Van den Block, G. Donker, L. Deliens, and B.D. Onwuteaka-Philipsen. 2011. Recognising patients who will die in the near future: A nationwide study via the Dutch sentinel netwrok of GPs. *British Journal of General Practice* 61 (587): 401–402.

Abela, J., and P. Mallia. 2016a. Maltese doctors: Views and experiences on end of life decisions and care. *Maltese Medical Journal* 28 (2): 16–26.

———. 2016b. Training in palliative care medicine and Maltese doctors: A cross-sectional survey. *Journal of the Malta College of Family Doctors* 5 (2): 13–19.

Atkinson, K., C. Jackson, and M. Rawlin. 2007. Competence and the quality framework. *Australian Family Physician* 36 (1/2): 24–27.

Ballatt, J., and P. Campling. 2013. *Intelligent kindness. Reforming the culture of health care.* London: RCPsych Publications.

Barclay, S., and A. Arthur. 2008. Place of death - how much does it matter? The priority is to improve end-of-life care in all settings. *British Journal of General Practice* 58 (549): 229–231.

Booth, B.J., and T. Snowdon. 2007. A quality framework for Australina general practice. *Australian Family Physician* 36 (1/2): 8–11.

Bradley, C. 2006. *General practice*. Edinburgh/London/New York/Oxford/Philadelphia/St. Louis/Sydney/Toronto: Elsevier.

Crane, M., and M. Wittink. 2005. Respecting end of life treatment preferences. *American Family Physician* 72 (7): 1263–1268.

Emery, J. 2013. End-of-life care: Identification, communication, training, and commissioning. *British Journal of General Practice* 63 (606): 6–7.

Field, David. 1998. Special not different: General practitioners' accounts of their Care of Dying People. *Social Science & Medicine* 46 (9): 1111–1120. https://doi.org/10.1016/S0277-9536(97)10041-7.

Flynn, J., B. Booth, and R. Portelli. 2007. Professionalism and the quality framework. *Australian Family Physician* 36: 16–19.

Kite, S. 2010. Advance care planning. *Clinical Medicine* 10 (3): 275–278.

Lang, F., and T. Quill. 2004. Making decisions with families at the end of life. *American Family Physician* 70 (4): 719–723.

Mahmoud, K., D. Munday, N. King, and J. Dale. 2008. Interprofessional relationships and communication in primary palliative care: Impact of the gold standards framework. *British Journal of General Practice, vol.* 58: 256–263.

National Palliative and End of Life Care Partnership. 2015. *Ambitions for palliative and end of life care: A national framework for lecal action 2015-2020.* National Palliative and End of Life Care Partnership.

Smith, G.P. 2001. Managing death: End-of-life charades and decisions. In *Aging: Decisions at the end of life*, ed. D.N. Weisstub, D.C. Thomasma, S. Gauthier, and G.F. Tomossy, 91–106. Dordrecht: Kluwer Academic Publishers.

Snowdon, T., J. Benson, and J. Proudfoot. 2007. Capacity and the quality framework. *Australian Family Physician* 36: 12–15.

Tan, S. 2007. Quality and general practice. *Australian Family Physician* 36 (1/2): 5–6.

Chapter 8
Team Approaches – How They Can Be Made to Work

Anthony Fiorini

Abstract A team approach is a recommended practice in the clinical management of all stages of a progressive illness. In this chapter, a geriatrician describes several practical steps he considers essential in ensuring an interprofessional team approach not only exists but also succeeds, even in end of life situations. These steps include the exposure of trainees to a team culture; the formulation of a mission statement which incorporates teamwork; the recruitment of the right members of different disciplines with the same ideas and commitment; the holding of regular clinical conferences to review and discuss patients. Examples are presented to highlight some potential problems which can arise, and advice is given on how they can be tackled or even avoided. Throughout this narrative, the author keeps emphasising that team approaches are a must, and can be made to work, not only to provide optimal clinical benefits to both patients and their relatives, but also to complement the job satisfaction of those working in such an environment.

Keywords Interprofessional team practice · Team culture · Mission statement · Team conference · Geriatric medicine

8.1 Introduction

On a recent family holiday, I visited a museum in Belfast, Northern Ireland, dedicated to the construction, launching, sinking and eventual recovery of that legendary and tragic ship, the Titanic. In the acknowledgments section of one of the museum's guidebooks, I read that the completion of such an impressive building and its exhibits, named the 'Belfast Titanic', was only achieved through a 'team effort' and surprisingly this statement was qualified in the text with a definition which was as

A. Fiorini (✉)
Clinical Chairperson of the Department of Geriatrics and a Consultant Geriatrician in the Department of Health, Msida, Malta
e-mail: anthony.fiorini@gov.mt

P. Mallia et al. (eds.), *Challenges to the Global Issue of End of Life Care*,
Advancing Global Bioethics 17, https://doi.org/10.1007/978-3-030-86386-9_8

follows: 'a group of people working collectively in the interests of a common goal' (Costecalde and Doherty 2012).

I like this definition, which is clear and concise. It contains the essential keywords and can easily be extrapolated to, and adapted for, a team working in health care practice – 'a group of professionals, representing different disciplines, working collectively in the interests of the patient'.

I can only surmise as to why the authors of the Titanic guidebook felt the need to define teamwork. They did not give an explanation. Maybe they kept being asked to amplify on their success. Certainly, in the institutions in which I practise geriatric medicine, I still keep finding myself having to remind colleagues and trainees about the importance of a team approach, what it actually entails and how it can be made to work. The invitation to write this chapter on this topic may also be a reflection on the need for such reminders.

There are of course many definitions of a health care team in the literature. Some of them can be quite a mouthful as they attempt to describe in detail the structure, the process and the expected outcome of team working, i.e. the three Donebedian categories which help evaluate the quality of care being given in a health service (St Leger et al. 1992). Such definitions are useful to explain theoretical concepts – they however do not give practical guidelines on how to make a team approach actually work.

Similarly, several published articles do list the principles of good team working, inserting such keywords as leadership, skill mix, vision, communication, training, respect and support (Nancarrow et al. 2013). Such described characteristics are obviously relevant and essential but again such principles that complement a definition are not necessarily a practical guide on how to set up a team and ensure it succeeds.

To complicate matters, discussions on teamwork can also become bogged down by uncertainty on terminology. Multidisciplinary, multiprofessional, interdisciplinary and interprofessional are the common terms used but whereas some may feel they all mean the same thing, and actually use these terms interchangeably or just stick to multidisciplinary, others insist on important differences and rightly so. Multidisciplinary and multiprofessional usually means people with different expertise focusing on the same patient but working in parallel, without formal arrangements for interaction. Interdisciplinary and interprofessional, on the other hand, implies that there is such a formal commitment for members to meet regularly and to work collectively (Beckingham 1997). There are now many teams in different health care subspecialties, and they tend to describe themselves as multidisciplinary, but that does not necessarily mean that they are all functioning in an interdisciplinary manner. If anything, in my experience, most members of such teams tend to function in parallel, with limited interaction.

There are also stated differences between the terms 'disciplinary' and 'professional', with the former including all members of a health care team, and the latter restricting members to a team of professionals only (Nancarrow et al. 2013). For the purpose of this article, I will be concentrating on, and using the term, 'interprofessionals' since this is the environment in which I work.

I do not claim to be an expert on the variety of team approaches, nor have I conducted some far-reaching research in this field. However, I can think of two main reasons why I have been invited to write this chapter. The first is that I am a practising consultant geriatrician and the core of the specialty of geriatrics consists of teamwork, thanks to the multifaceted and inter-related problems a frail older person might face. The second reason for this invitation is that I am considered a bit of a pioneer in the country where I still practise, since I introduced and helped set up the specialty of geriatrics from scratch, and to ensure it succeeded, I had to concomitantly help initiate a team concept and approach, which was another novelty then. As further evidence on my ability to discuss, and advise on this subject, I can also state that way back in the year 1995, I was part of a group organising a conference on geriatrics in Malta – we called the conference 'Developing inter-professional practice in the care of older persons' (Fiorini and Muscat 1995), certainly new terms at that time.

Whilst discussing teamwork, as a practising geriatrician, I can also comment on end of life situations. Specialists in geriatric medicine are able to competently manage the whole spectrum of disease stages through which their patients pass, from the initial and usually acute and rehabilitative aspects, through the reversible dips in health and function caused by medical complications, right up to the palliative and terminal phases. Their holistic role is emphasised in definitions of 'Geriatrics' such as the one compiled by the European Union of Medical Specialists (2008) which also mentions within 'a multidisciplinary team setting'. Most of the illnesses geriatricians deal with are chronic and progressive. They are therefore actively involved in end of life care on a daily basis, whether in a hospital, or in a long-term care institution, or even in the community. There is no doubt that team working is essential in all three environments, and in all stages of a progressive illness, in order for patients and their relatives to feel they have derived the optimal benefit from the clinical care possible.

This chapter therefore focuses on how to compose a team representing a number of different disciplines i.e. the structure, and ensure all members practise in an inter-professional collective manner, i.e. the process, for the benefit of the patient i.e. the expected outcome. It describes a number of practical steps which, in my opinion and based on my clinical experiences, are essential in order to ensure that teamwork succeeds. They can be applied to any clinical scenario, including end of life care. I will be describing both the successes and the frustrations, peppering my narrative with appropriate examples. I will endeavour to mix academia with everyday hands on clinical practice, but with an emphasis on the latter.

I hope readers will find this chapter useful not only to increase their knowledge and encourage further reading, but also to help them review and maybe change the way they work, and even convince others about the benefits. After all, this is how team practice begins.

8.2 Experiencing a Team Culture

Being brought up, and having the experience of working and being trained in an everyday hands-on team culture is, in my opinion, the first essential step in helping to make a team approach succeed.

I got to know all about teamwork as a trainee in the specialty of geriatric medicine in the United Kingdom, in the nineteen eighties, when it was already well established there. So it certainly is not a relatively new or recent concept. I did not attend any lectures or tutorials or workshops on the subject, there were none then, but as was the norm at that time, I learnt by observing my mentors and participating in the team conferences on ward rounds and in the day hospital. Eventually I was allowed, and learnt how, to conduct them myself.

I can still recall being at first incredulous, and then astonished, whilst observing how a group of professionals of different disciplines could find the time to sit down and discuss in detail each and every patient for whom they were responsible, and how my consultant would take the same amount of time to listen to the feedback of all present and reach a common decision. There were occasions when my consultant had to correct and change his initial assessment and conclusions, based on the opinions of the other members of the team. Most times, relatives, and even the patients themselves, were invited to attend these meetings.

I was hooked. I was converted from a 'know it all and can do it all myself' yuppie doctor to a team player and was gradually encouraged to develop my skills in such an environment. I eventually just carried the baton to a different country, helping to set up such similar concepts, and the way of practice, in Malta.

I was recently reminded how disruptive a new member of a team can be, if not brought up and trained in such an interprofessional culture and environment. Problems surfaced when a service that provided therapy for a selective group of patients with neurological problems was relocated to the hospital where the department of geriatric medicine was mainly based. As a result, a number of therapists were also transferred and had to join the system of team working that had been in operation for a good number of years. Unfortunately, it quickly became obvious that these therapists had no experience and no inkling of what interprofessional practice meant, and even worse, being used to working alone and in parallel with other disciplines, refused to adapt and be bound by the code of conduct that governed such a team. One particular therapist kept meeting relatives of patients on his own, providing them with his plan of treatment and discharge options, whilst stating he was too busy to attend ward round conferences. Of course, this unilateral mode of working had to be stopped but whilst it lasted it precipitated arguments and frustrations amongst other team members, with patients and relatives bewildered at receiving different and even contradictory information.

I am still involved in giving lectures on teams and team working. For both undergraduates and postgraduates, I used to drag representatives of other disciplines with me to participate in the presentation and for students to see a team on stage. Whilst such a 'class-room' demonstration helps to explain concepts, it can never, and does not, replicate or replace a team meeting occurring live on site. Similarly, so called team building exercises have become the norm in many organisations. Such activities, whilst encouraging camaraderie and helping to overcome professional barriers, certainly do not replicate a team conference at a clinical level.

Students and trainees of all clinical disciplines must therefore be brought up in a team culture. It must be ingrained in their DNA as early as possible. Didactic teaching helps to set the ball rolling but nothing beats observing and participating in a team meeting conducted by committed and experienced professionals, in an interdisciplinary manner, at the workplace.

8.3 Ownership and Mission Statements

For team practice to work and succeed there must be an agreement with the authorities in management. If anything, health service managers should be expected to not only encourage and facilitate such clinical practice, but to also come up with the idea in the first place! Even better, management itself should be seen to be practising in such an identical manner.

In the hospital I helped set up, which concentrated mainly on the comprehensive assessment and rehabilitation of ill older persons, I was lucky enough to be actively involved not only at a clinical level but also in management issues. I was surrounded by other like-minded determined individuals, all working closely on a daily basis, with both clinical and management responsibilities. We were given a relatively free reign by higher authorities and since we started completely from scratch, even in the recruitment and training of staff, we were able to introduce and maintain our ideas and standards, including the introduction of interprofessional work practices.

A well-known, successful and highly respective Scottish football personality once stated that you must have ownership and control to ensure your vision succeeds (Meek and Tyrrell 2011). How true this statement is. Later experiences showed that whenever authorities and managers changed to those imposing unilateral control and issuing instructions without prior discussion, team practice, even at a clinical level suffered and was in danger of collapsing.

For teamwork to succeed, the keywords ‘team’ and ‘practice’ must be inserted in the mission statement of the health organisation, for all to see and follow. For example, the mission statement compiled for the hospital I worked in purposely emphasised such a process ‘........ staff will work with patients and their carers, in an interdisciplinary team approach within a high-quality atmosphere, conducive to learning and to continual development, which promotes rehabilitation for the older persons to regain maximal independence for reintegration into society’.

I used to think that mission statements were somewhat woolly and tedious to compile. For example, it took the team several sessions of a few hours each to come up with the one I just quoted. But if it genuinely describes the structure, process and outcome of the organisation and if it is religiously followed, or allowed to be pursued, then the effort is well worth the while. The wording and font size of this mission statement was magnified and framed and placed in a prominent place in the entrance lobby of the hospital. So many people would stop to read it and approve. Members of staff would proudly glance at it when arriving for work, a reminder of the quality care given by working in such a manner.

Just like my conversion from a single independent trainee doctor to working as part of a team, so was my opinion of mission statements similarly changed. I therefore recommend that every organisation should compile its own statement, ensuring that the words interdisciplinary or interprofessional are added if teamwork is practised in that manner, and insist that it is on show in a prominent position to remind everybody how the organisation works and why it succeeds.

Just like the authors of the Belfast Titanic guide felt the need to define 'team effort', so must an organisation, even one providing end of life care, continuously strive to inform and remind staff on how they should be working.

8.4 Recruiting the Right Members

For a team to function in an interprofessional manner not only must there be the right skill mix of members to cover a comprehensive assessment and management plan, but such members must also believe, and want to work, in a team environment.

Unfortunately, many discipline representatives have not been trained, or do not have the right experience of working in such environments, as already mentioned. This situation becomes more obvious whenever there is a rotation of staff. For example, therapists might regularly rotate from one ward to another, or from one institution to another as part of their training or to allow them to obtain a wider range of clinical experience. For many, this placement might be their first ever contact with a team functioning in an efficient interprofessional manner. If they happen to be the only representatives of a particular core discipline, then the team dynamics might suffer because of their lack of experience, since all members are dependent on each other in order to provide an efficient and quality service.

Such trainees might become hooked on team working, like I had become at their stage, but on many occasions when they have settled in and have overcome their shyness and are contributing as wanted, they are moved on to pastures new in other institutions. Sometimes of course, on the other hand, it is a relief to see a team member who has not settled in, or contributed, move on. But the wheat and the chaff tend to rotate together and usually at too short a notice.

I therefore recommend that trainees should not be left alone as the sole representative of a discipline in a team. A more senior established member, keen and knowledgeable on interprofessional team working, should also always be present. But I must admit that a lack of human resources might not allow this ideal situation to happen on a regular basis.

Apart from the problem of inexperienced staff trying to fit into an established team, I can think of two other situations where staff problems can interfere with proper team working. The first is a serious one, where a representative of a profession openly declares that he or she does not believe in working in an interprofessional manner, and prefers to, and does assess and manage patients alone, without ever giving any feedback. I gave an example of such a situation earlier in this narrative, to demonstrate that it can happen – such individuals should be immediately transferred out of the unit.

The second situation is when a team exists but the leader, usually a doctor, even at a consultant level, prefers to, and does, function by not only conducting the orchestra but also by attempting to play all the instruments (Tallis 1990), instructing other disciplines on what to do, what interventions to carry out, and how to manage a patient, even taking unilateral decisions and informing team members afterwards. Such individuals should be politely reminded about the proper way the team should function and how it should be led. Just as the authors of the Titanic guidebook felt the need to define teamwork, such leaders should also be made aware of such a definition and should be shown again the mission statement of the institution.

8.5 The Team Conference

I firmly believe that the team meeting, also called the conference, remains the crux of proper team working. This conference is a must and should be conducted on a regular weekly basis, more often if required. It must be held in a quiet room, around a table, with all core members of the team present. I do not think that patients and their relatives should be there for all the discussions, but they should be invited in at some stage, if and when appropriate. Certainly, in end of life situations they will have to be involved.

A regular conference, held in such surroundings, demonstrates that proper interprofessional practice is taking place. Even after a ward round, no matter how long it has been, team members should then sit around a table and again present and discuss every patient and reach a common decision, on all relevant aspects. A conference is a symbol that communication and collaboration, amongst members, is taking place. A nice cup of tea or mug of coffee for everyone, including students, coupled with a packet of fresh biscuits, will help the dialogue considerably. And one of the advantages of a rotation of staff is that such individuals might even turn up for their last conference with a tasty cake to be shared by all, in an interdisciplinary manner of course!

I presently mainly work in two separate institutions, dealing with frail older persons in both. But whereas one of these institutions encourages team working by providing a conference room on each ward, the other, on the other hand, even while undergoing an extensive refurbishment programme, prefers to emphasise the creation of more beds, forgoing space necessary for a private and quiet team meeting. Any team discussions in this second institution have to take place whilst standing on a ward round, with such a process being far from ideal, tending to occur in a potentially noisy environment, lacking privacy and being overall less thorough and efficient. Similarly, I know of consultants who still prefer to conduct a team discussion at the bedside even though a conference room is available. Again, in my opinion, such processes are not conducive to proper interprofessional practice.

Another reason why sitting round a table is essential is the need for documentation. Executive style summaries of discussions and decisions have to be written in each patient's file in a legible and easy to understand manner. The entries will have to be read by all members of the team. Documentation carried out at the bedside tends to be hurried, may be difficult to read and may miss out on important points. I also feel that the person leading the discussion should write and summarize. That way, again, decisions get properly documented and understood. Certainly, whenever I am leading a team conference at a clinical level, I insist and ensure I do all the writing.

I am sounding old fashioned, talking about writing. I am aware and appreciate that some institutions have now switched to computerised documentation but whatever medium is used, the principle, in my eyes, remains the same – the leader should document.

Obviously, a team conference takes time and effort. It should take place directly after a ward round when assessments, findings, ideas and management plans are still fresh and not later on at the end of the day or even worse on another day. And the day of the week and the time of the conference should be kept regular and constant to allow individual members of the team to plan their work accordingly. Even if some members of the team join the ward round, the conference should still take place with these same members present.

In the institution I had helped set up, an assessment and rehabilitation hospital for older people called Zammit Clapp Hospital where interprofessional practice was introduced into Malta and whose mission statement I quoted earlier, a postgraduate student was granted permission to carry out fieldwork for her thesis to establish whether team work was actually being carried out (Buttigieg 2002). Whilst in her conclusions she had established that the hospital was unique at that time in adopting and successfully using an interdisciplinary team practice, even describing the hospital as a model of best practice, the author had interestingly demonstrated and noted that the ward round I led had lasted two and a half hours whilst the conference had lasted for a further 2 h. This means that the time spent assessing and discussing patients had nearly doubled because of the team conference. All team members have to know this and have to accordingly plan for the conference and allocate time to attend and participate regularly and religiously, if interprofessional practice is to work properly.

In a realistic world, with a lack of human resources, where a team member is given the task of working in more than one ward, it might be tempting for that individual to avoid attending conferences, feeling that 2 h could be better utilised elsewhere. Such reasoning should never be accepted. Similarly, interprofessional team practices can be threatened by the development of sub-specialisation. For example, one tissue viability nurse might have to cover the whole hospital and will not attend any conferences – but just leaving instructions on management is not conducive to team practicing. In one of the hospitals I am presently working in, a continence nurse has just been appointed. It dawned on me that a decision to remove the catheter of a patient, the yes, when and how, could now not be decided in the conference because the sub-specialty nurse was not present, again interrupting teamwork.

One might argue that such specialised nurses, who focus on a specific clinical problem, are not core members of a team and need not be present or involved in all decisions affecting a particular patient but, in my experience, their absence at a conference interferes with holistic care and hence optimal team working. At least they should be present when the patient is being discussed – their instructions might have had a bearing on how other disciplines were managing the patient.

The same argument holds for other disciplines such as dieticians, pharmacists and speech therapists. Many frail older persons will be on multiple medications and have multiple problems including nutrition and swallowing concerns. In end of life care, decisions have to be made on what medication needs to be stopped or started, on whether tube feeding needs to be considered and on whether their diet needs to be restricted or liberated. Such complex issues have to be discussed in the presence of all team members. In my experience, difficulties encountered in team working at end of life issues have nearly always focused on medication and nutrition because of unilateral decisions, as I will discuss further in the next section of this chapter.

Although I am emphasising that all those professional staff actively involved in the decision making on the care and management of a patient should be present for the conference, on the other hand, the total number of members participating should be kept manageable to allow the team to function in an efficient manner. I am not aware of any recommended maximum or even minimum numbers for a conference – it depends on the service being given and how many core members there are. But certainly, in a hospital, one conference should concentrate on one ward. I once had to briefly work in a geriatrics hospital in the United Kingdom when, at that time, there was just one massive conference for all wards. This meant that the meeting room was too crowded and busy, with staff from several wards present, having to listen to discussions about other patients that did not concern them. Such a conference lacked focus. This method of working was chosen by the hospital to accommodate staff, such as doctors, who were responsible for patients scattered in several wards, but it certainly was not conducive to interprofessional practice. There was always a continuous murmur in the room as members present talked amongst themselves waiting for their patients to be discussed and I can imagine today many fiddling with their mobile phones, if such a type of conference still took place – irritated, I would be unable to concentrate and lead such a meeting.

So far, I have concentrated on hospitals, since this is the environment I am used to working in. However, I am also aware that team care and team practices take place in community settings, in patients' own houses or in care homes. More recently, doctors working in the Department of Geriatric Medicine I form part of, started increasing their input in the community and I again had to appreciate the difficulties a team might face when trying to meet in such circumstances. Individual discipline representatives tend to visit patients on their own, continually travelling from one site to another. Still, even in such situations, where patients are receiving input from more than one discipline, the case manager has to ensure that team conferences take place at a site and time convenient for all, having the necessary facilities where to sit down and discuss quietly. It can certainly take place in a care home, with the participation of the client and relative when necessary. A team member, such as a social worker, can act as their advocate at a team meeting if, for example, the patient and relative are living in their own home and cannot travel to another site.

I have concentrated mainly on the conference in this chapter on team working because I want to keep emphasising its importance. I firmly believe that it is the most important element of interprofessional practice. It ensures communication and collaboration, allowing discussions and common decisions to take place on a regular basis, all of which are essential ingredients for a model of best practice. However, problems can still occasionally arise even when such meetings are regularly taking place, as is discussed in the next section.

8.6 Team Problems at End of Life

The problems I have encountered in clinical issues at end of life can be attributed to either a lack of communication or to a lack of agreement within a team. The involvement of relatives is also of critical importance at this stage of care, as they can also try and influence clinical decisions.

A lack of communication usually occurs when an individual team member, or one discipline, decides to take unilateral action without prior discussion. The incidents I recall, which involved patients I was responsible for, mainly concentrated on whether tube feeding should be started or even stopped, as the following brief examples will show.

One older patient who presented with a sudden onset of a hemiplegia was found to have a large inoperable brain tumour on a CT brain scan, rather than a stroke. As the patient deteriorated, entering a coma because of increasing intracranial pressure, despite prescribing medication to combat this added complication, the nurses on the ward decided to insert a nasogastric tube to facilitate feeding, and the administration of other medications, without prior team discussion or the involvement of relatives. As a result, the patient's life was unnecessarily prolonged by a few weeks and the inevitable postponed.

More recently, a bedbound patient with advanced Parkinson's disease, who was a resident in a long-term care facility and who was having swallowing difficulties, also had a nasogastric tube inserted, at the insistence of relative who happened to be a nurse by profession, working in another institution. The team discussion and decision in a prior ward round had opted to avoid this procedure for the time being, with the plan being to alter the consistency of the food further, to facilitate intake, and to hold a meeting with her relatives to discuss her further management. However, at the insistence of her son, a nurse on the ward had to take the initiative and insert a tube without allowing the team to meet again to discuss the issue further.

A similar situation occurred in the same long-term facility, involving a patient's guardian and a senior resident doctor, who this time decided to remove a nasogastric tube. A very frail patient with multiple co-morbidities, limb contractures and pressure ulcers, was transferred to the institution from the acute general hospital. The doctor who assessed her felt that she was in too much discomfort, whilst anticipating she only had a few days or weeks to live. He therefore decided to start morphine and administer it via a subcutaneous pump and at the same time stop all other futile medications and even remove the nasogastric tube. Whilst his assessment and prognosis proved correct, his actions were too quick, without consulting other members of the team or the patient's relatives. As a result, the patient's guardian insisted that the tube feeding be recommenced whilst even the nurses on the ward were uncomfortable with the sudden withdrawal of nutrition and medications.

This last case scenario raises several points on problems that may arise at end of life, even when trying to work as a team. The first demonstrates the importance of always involving relatives at this stage in the planned clinical management. The second point raised shows how different professional members of a team might have different views about if and when to withhold or withdraw treatment. Although learned bodies publish guidelines on such situations, I have learned to be cautious on such a delicate matter and tend to manage patients after gauging the mood and feelings of other team members, especially nurses who might have difficulties letting go. The third point concerns the method of handover from one institution to another. Geriatricians tend to inherit patients from other firms and teams who might have already made difficult, and even contentious, clinical decisions. The times I have had to face a new patient on a ward round replete with clinical intricacies and dilemmas, based on previous decisions I was not part of, are too numerous to count. Prior communication from the teams looking after such a patient, or from the gate keeper who accepted and arranged the transfer, is essential and expected, but not always carried out. And the final point, therefore, concerns the need to allow a patient to settle in a new environment, giving ample time to the members of the team to properly assess a new arrival and discuss the identified issues, even talking to relatives, before making decisions, especially difficult ones such as the removal of a feeding tube, or stopping futile treatment.

Such experiences are again a reminder that there should be an individualised rather than a 'one glove fits all' clinical approach (Hodgkinson et al. 2016). Older patients and their relatives have different backgrounds, beliefs, needs and desires and should be managed appropriately. This is another reason why a interprofessional team approach is necessary, even in end of life situations.

8.7 Conclusions

In this chapter, I have attempted to present and discuss the subject of how to make team approaches work. I have been as practical as possible by offering advice based on my clinical experiences in geriatric medicine, a specialty in which team working is a must, as well as on my previous position of forming part of a group who successfully introduced and developed interprofessional team working from scratch in Malta, in a hospital providing hands on care to frail older people.

I have mentioned and discussed several essential ingredients which, in my opinion, are necessary to ensure team working is built on sound foundations, including the formulation of a relevant mission statement, the feeling of ownership, the exposure of trainees to such an environment, the recruitment of the right staff and the importance of a regular team conference. Out of these five ingredients, the team conference held in a quiet, private and unrushed environment remains, in my opinion, the most essential as it ensures that communication and collaboration are maintained on a frequent and regular basis.

I do not feel that such an interprofessional approach is difficult to achieve. It however does require a continuous commitment and it does take up more time of an already busy working schedule. There must, of course, be the common will of several like minded individuals, representing several disciplines, to be able to work in this manner.

Overall, I have discussed general or generic principles of team working but these are also relevant to end of life scenarios. I have used this stage of a disease to give some examples of how clinical problems can still surface, even when professional representatives of different disciplines are working as a team, but I purposely did not go into further details on the management of patients in end of life situations, and the other problems and dilemmas that may arise at this stage, since this was not my remit and are competently tackled by other authors in other chapters of this book.

Many lessons were learned from the sinking of the Titanic, over a 100 years ago. Subsequent boards of inquiry emphasised the importance of better ship designs, of more efficient and effective crews and of ensuring the safety of all passengers, echoing again the Donebedian categories of structure, process and outcome when evaluating the quality of a health service. A more recent guidebook of the Belfast museum dedicated to the history of this ship, has added another recommendation relevant to health care professionals, a reminder of the benefits that will be reaped if a group of different disciplines work collectively in the interests of a common goal. I hope I have been as convincing in explaining the need for a team approach and how it can be made to succeed, even in end of life care, not only for the good of all patients and their relatives, but also for the job satisfaction of those working in such an environment.

References

Beckingham, A.C. 1997. *BOLD* 7 (2): 17–23.

Buttigieg, S. 2002. *Teamwork in health care delivery – A case study of a Maltese geriatric hospital.* MBA. University of Malta.

Costecalde, C., and J.P. Doherty. 2012. *Titanic Belfast souvenir guide*. Ireland: Booklink, Acknowledgements.

European Union of Medical Specialists Geriatrics Section. 2008. *Definition of geriatrics*. https://uemsgeriatricmedicine.org/www/land/definition/english.asp. Accessed 22 Jan 2019.

Fiorini, A., and H. Muscat. 1995. DIPCOP: Developing inter-professional practice in the care of older persons. *Malta Medical Journal* VII (2): 15.

Hodgkinson, S., J. Ruegger, A. Field-Smith, S. Latchem, and S.H. Ahmedzai. 2016. Care of dying adults in the last days of life. *Clinical Medicine* 16 (3): 254–258.
Meek, D., and T. Tyrrell. 2011. *Sir Alex Ferguson*, 18. UK: Simon and Schuster.
Nancarrow, S.A., A. Booth, S. Ariss, T. Smith, P. Enderby, and A. Roots. 2013. Ten principles of good interdisciplinary team work. *Hum Resources Health*. [online] http://www.human-resources-health.com/content/11/1/19 Accessed 13 Dec 2018.
St Leger, A.S., H. Schnieden, and J.P. Walsworth-Bell. 1992. *Evaluating health services effectiveness*, 2–3. Milton Keynes: Open University Press.
Tallis, R. 1990. *Medical rehabilitation*. Update in Geriatric Medicine, Malta.

Chapter 9
Communication and Conflict Resolution – Managing Conversations. A Culturally Sensitive Model

Sarah Cox

Abstract Conflict can arise around care at the end of life. This is understandable as families face the death of a loved one. There may be disagreement between the health care professionals' view and the wishes of the family or patient. Communication can compound disagreement, with high levels of emotional investment, lack of trust and the individuals involved defending their views. This may lead to increased polarisation and increased conflict and is not helpful for the care of the patient in the middle of all this. Communication can also be the means to reduce conflict and resolve differences in end of life care. The chapter discusses how good communication skills can help to minimise and manage conflict.

Keywords Communication · Conflict · Consensus · Empathy · Trust

9.1 Introduction

Most of the time we communicate without stopping to consider the way we do it and the words we use, and most of the time this is not a problem. However, at the end of life there are difficult conversations health professionals need to have which require more thought. These conversations can have a lasting negative impact on the recipients and may make further discussions harder. Health professionals can feel unprepared and distressed by the sense they have been the cause of sadness. As a result, these conversations may be avoided. This can result in patients being poorly informed about the length and likely course of their lives and being unable to prepare or plan for what is to come. Patients and families may be unwilling to accept the news of treatment failure, or a short prognosis and this can lead to conflict, with loss of trust and breakdown in the relationship between the patient and family and the clinical team.

S. Cox (✉)
Chelsea and Westminster Hospital, London, UK
e-mail: sarah.cox39@nhs.net

P. Mallia et al. (eds.), *Challenges to the Global Issue of End of Life Care*, Advancing Global Bioethics 17, https://doi.org/10.1007/978-3-030-86386-9_9

This chapter presents an overview of communication around end of life care issues, taking a global view and challenging some entrenched ideas. First, the types of situations in which these conversations might arise are described, together with the problems they are associated with and how to recognise them. The evidence of the impact of end of life care conversations supports the need for training but we continue to find them difficult and the reasons for this are explored. Practical tips and pitfalls of conversations are considered including an appropriate environment, how to open the conversation, and what to look out for. It is also important to understand how to end conversations and to think about follow up afterwards. Issues to think about at the end and after the conversation are reviewed. Ways of managing conflict are discussed and resolving differences are discussed. Global perspectives are explored throughout to ensure this chapter has relevance in different cultures.

1. Which conversations are we talking about and when should we have them?

Challenging conversations at the end of life are often described as "breaking bad news" and many are around the subject of imparting new and negative information. However, "breaking bad news" does not describe all of the issues requiring expert communication at the end of life. Also, the term suggests that the conversation is a one time and perhaps a one-sided event which may not be the most helpful way to consider what should be a sensitive, ongoing and two-way discussion.

In the course of life-limiting illnesses, Western cultures hold that it is important to offer a discussion with patients to ensure they understand what the future might hold. This opens the possibility of making informed choices about future treatment, including, for some, choosing not to have some investigations or interventions (see Chaps. 7 and 10). Picking the right time for this conversation is tricky; there are often no "milestone" investigations to prompt it and the disease progression and prognosis may be very uncertain (Barclay and Maher 2010). It therefore relies heavily on skilled professionals to the pick the right time to offer this conversation. It is perhaps not surprising that the evidence is that these conversations are not happening as often as they should (Fawole et al. 2013; Haidet et al. 1998; SUPPORT Principle Investigators 1995).

Perhaps the most frequent challenging conversation occurs when there is new information about a life-limiting condition to give to a patient or those close to them. This may be a new diagnosis of cancer, or progression or recurrence of a disease that can no longer be cured or failure to respond to treatment after a catastrophic event such as cardiac arrest or trauma.

In the case of cancer there may be investigations which have been undertaken which clearly prompt the conversation at a particular time. For sudden events where the patient does not die immediately but soon afterwards, the conversation is also defined in time by the realisation of the healthcare team that treatment is not working.

The information that a patient is in the last days or weeks of life is important to discuss with them if possible and they wish it, and with their relatives. The healthcare team may wish to limit intervention or set a ceiling on the patient's treatment as they consider it to be futile. This is sometimes a source of conflict, particularly between the health professional and the relative. Families may reject the assessment of the doctors even when the patient is in their last hours or days. The family may be desperately clinging to their loved one, unable to accept the futility of further treatment. In some religions, only God can decide what will happen in the future. A doctor making a pronouncement of the likelihood of impending death is likely to be rejected or challenged for this reason.

In each of these situations, it is usually the healthcare professionals that needs to identify that the patient may have limited life left, in order to initiate the conversation. Doctors, nurses and therapists will vary in their ability to recognise when a patient is at the end of their life. Their access to specific education around end of life care but also their culture and personal values will influence how ready they are to consider it.

2. What are we aiming for?

Good communication results in an informed patient who can engage in decision making. In many cultures the patient would then decide who they wish to be informed, and their wishes would be respected. The aim in these systems is to give the patient as much information as is available so they can understand the options and make informed choices about the future (Teno et al. 2001). Knowing you have a limited prognosis might change your decision-making about healthcare but also about how you relate to family, what you choose to do about work, travel and other aspects of home life too. Good communication can also have other benefits for the patient such as improved emotional and physical health (Stewart 1995).

However, these conversations are not happening in many cultures. In Iran, there is no legal requirement to inform patients of their diagnosis. There are privacy laws which would support patients being told first, but the usual practice is to inform the family first (Scheldt et al. 2017). In Canada, 70% of elderly patients admitted to hospital have thought about end of life care issues but only 30% had discussed their wishes with healthcare professionals (Heyland et al. 2013). Patients assume that health professionals will initiate these conversations, whilst clinicians wait for patients to ask (Almack et al. 2012). This results in a stand-off where the communication may not be started by ether party.

In other cultures, patients and their families may not want or expect negative information to be shared with them (Blackhall et al. 1995; Hunt 1998). Individual autonomy may be of less importance in some cultures than others and cultural values are critical to holistic care. For instance, information about prognosis is wanted by 88% of patients in Turkey but only 52% of patients in Pakistan (Rosenberg et al. 2017). Families may expect bad news to be told to them first and for them to choose how or whether to pass this on to the patient. In some cultures, women would expect that medical information would be told to their husband or father, and only selectively relayed to them.

Where family members request that a patient is not given bad news, it is usually because the family (or the health professional) feels the patient would be badly affected by it, even to the extent that they might die more quickly (Zhang and Siminoff 2003). The cultural belief is that it is the role of the family to take the burden of decision-making to relieve the suffering of the patient (Koenig and Gates-Williams 1995). This underlines the importance of understanding the patient and family's views about the illness and further information, and to personalise these conversations rather than having a "one size fits all" approach.

Where the health professional and patient speak different languages, a family member is sometimes a convenient translator. However, an interpreter may be more appropriate if the aim is to ensure the patient's wishes for information are met.

A universal aim of initiating end of life conversations could therefore be to gain a better understanding of what the patients knows and what information they may wish to have, rather than aiming for full disclosure of all the medical news.

3. Why are these conversations difficult?

Even the most experienced of communicators may pause before having a conversation about end of life care. Some of this relates to a reluctance on the part of the professional to cause distress. It is difficult for most people deliberately to cause harm to another person, and healthcare professionals, who may have chosen the profession for the opportunity to do good, may find it even harder. Doctors struggle to use the word "dying" and may try to soften the impact of the words by using softer language such as "seriously ill" or "very poorly".

Clinicians may not wish to start a conversation in which they may be asked questions they cannot answer such as how long a patient has left to live (Brighton and Bristowe 2016).

Individual professionals may fear saying the wrong thing and making a bad situation worse. They may lack confidence or feel they have insufficient knowledge or skill. They may understand the importance of good, sensitive skilled communication but fear that they do not have enough training or time (Almack et al. 2012).

In fact, sensitive communication can be carried out as a series of smaller discussions. Education and development in communication is essential to improve the ability of all professionals to initiate and carry out conversations around end of life care issues. Communication skills continue to develop with experience and senior professionals also benefit from reflection and refinement of their skills.

Another barrier to initiating end of life conversations is the fear of taking away hope and the damage this may cause (Almack et al. 2012). In fact, there is some evidence that sensitive communication can enhance patients' ability to be hopeful (Davison and Simpson 2006). It seems we need to distinguish different types of hope, not all of which are death-denying, but rather affirm life for whatever time is left (Eliot and Olver 2009).

There may be a reluctance to share bad news on the part of the professional, or a concern that sharing the information would be culturally insensitive to the patient or family. Potential cultural barriers include language barriers, patients and families not trusting health professionals, possibly due to previous real or perceived discrimination, and religious or cultural beliefs about death and dying (Periyakoil et al. 2015). Examples of this include discussing life-limiting disease with patients whose religion suggests that only God can dictate what will happen to them in the future and therefore it may be consider disrespectful or inappropriate for a health professional to suggest they know what the future holds (Koenig and Gates-Williams 1995).

There is some evidence that there is cultural change in some countries with practices moving closer to full disclosure. In Lebanon, a law requiring informed consent was passed in 2004. The percentage of Lebanese physicians reporting full disclosure has changed from 47% in 1998 to 99% in 2007 (Rosenberg et al. 2017).

Professionals may be concerned about the strong emotional reactions that will naturally occur when end of life care issues are discussed. Sadness, grief, despondency, disbelief and anger may all be experienced and expressed by the patient. It may be uncomfortable for the health professional to witness the patient feeling these strong emotions. They may be able to react naturally in their private life to those around them who are distressed or upset, but they may be unsure how to react in their professional life. They may wish to offer comfort but fear being contaminated by the emotional impact of the patient's illness. Health professionals tend to be poorly prepared in their training to deal with expressions of emotion and can feel inadequate as a result.

4. What are potential sources of conflict in end of life communication?

When a patient is in the last year, or months or days of life, conversations between clinicians, the patient and the family are often emotionally difficult. The clinician is giving information they wish they didn't have to give, the patient wishes it wasn't true and the family may be looking for any source of hope, even if this means rejecting the opinion of the clinician.

Over a long illness patients and families may have met a huge number of healthcare professionals, and not all these encounters will have been perfect. There may have been an erosion of trust in clinicians as a result (Crawley et al. 2002). The patient and family may have searched for alternative treatments for their illness once pronounced incurable by their traditional healthcare team. They may have been encouraged to ignore the advice of traditional professionals, with a further reduction in trust.

In some cultures, we are seeing a general increased questioning of doctors, which whilst healthy to a degree, can also lead to increased conflict. The expectations of what healthcare can achieve are rising (Hoffmann and Del Mar 2015). There are frequent stories in the news about the advances of medicine with new technologies, drugs or therapies, but very little about the limitations of medicine. Even in cultures where there is more open discussion around end of life care, society generally remains rather death-denying. It is therefore difficult for patients and families to accept when professionals claim they cannot make an illness better.

Conflict may arise where the clinical team and patient hold different religious, cultural or moral beliefs. The judgement about whether a patient is dying may seem to be a clinical one to a doctor, when the same question may seem a deeply religious one to some patients and families. Patients and families who believe in the sanctity of life may view attempts to discuss limitation of treatment as deeply wrong (Koenig and Gates-Williams 1995). Unless there is understanding of, and allowance for these two very different perspectives, conflict is possible. Healthcare teams sometimes wish to limit invasive treatment which they consider futile in order to "do no harm". This ethical perspective may be at odds with certain views or cultures who hold life to be precious "at all costs" and reject the importance of burden as an argument to limiting treatment.

When a patient is unable to be involved in making decisions about their healthcare, a decision must be made in their best interests. The healthcare team will have a view based on their experience of similar patients and understanding of what the future may hold, together with a value judgement of the patient's quality of life. This is likely to be influenced by the professional's own values and beliefs (Stewart et al. 1999). The family will have their own view of what is best for the patient and this may be driven by selfish motives but also by what they know of the patient. It is important to remember that the family are our best way of understanding the view of the patient (Heyland et al. 2013). In these situations, the professional needs to understand all of these perspectives to support a good decision being reached with consensus (Teno et al. 1995).

Clinicians may have to make decisions based on the good of society rather than the good of the individual. Availability of resources, for instance of transplant organs, may limit possible treatments for an individual and this will be difficult to accept for that individual and their family. Where there is also rationing through limited funding for a treatment that the patient and family believe would be life-prolonging, this can also be a source of conflict.

Communication with patients and families can be made more difficult where there are different views of what should happen within the family. Sometimes family members feel very differently about what is right for the patient because they have different values and beliefs, sometimes it is an expression of a long-lasting family feud. Recognition of this and communication with all parties together is essential.

Conflict can arise from inconsistent messages from the healthcare team. When there is already mistrust, communication that seems contradictory is incredibly challenging for patients and families, worsening mistrust and increasing the likelihood of conflict. This can easily arise where different teams are involved in the care of a patient, but also where different team members have different views of what is happening, or what should happen. Careful communication between team members is therefore also essential.

5. Why is the right amount of healthcare information at the end of life?

The Western perspective is that patients need information about their health in order to make informed choices about healthcare decisions. This is true of all healthcare decisions, not just at the end of life. However, understanding that they are at the end of life will allow a patient to make decisions not just about healthcare decisions but also about how they live the rest of their lives and how they prepare themselves and those around them for their death (Teno et al. 2001). The knowledge gives them the opportunity to do things that are really important to them before they die (such as getting married), to prepare financially (for instance writing a will), to prepare family and friends emotionally (for instance to create memories for young children in the form of letters and videos), and to heal fractured relationships with family and friends. It also helps them to make decisions about where they would like their care to be and how much medical intervention they want.

In Chinese and Tibetan cultures, recognising dying is also important to enable the patient to be at home with their family. However, the goals of care may be quite different, with the focus on maintaining a clear mind and continuing to treat the source of the illness, rather than on symptom control (Hsieh and Wang 2012).

For some patients, understanding why they are not getting better can be a source of relief. It may seem counterintuitive, but many patients feel less distressed by news that their illness is incurable than they do living with deterioration and uncertainty about the cause. It is also important in maintaining a relationship of trust with healthcare professionals if their requests for honest information are met with honesty. Conflict can arise in this case if a patient wants information and the family does not want them burdened by it.

Not all patients wish to be told they are dying or to understand everything about their disease and its likely progression (Barclay and Maher 2010). Giving information that a patient is not ready to deal with can result in negative consequences for them, and distress and anger from the family. The role of the healthcare professional, therefore, is to find out what information the patient wants and is ready to deal with. It is perfectly acceptable to withhold information from a patient if they have been offered it and make it clear they do not wish to hear it. There should be further ongoing offers of information or answers to questions as patients may subsequently change their mind about the information they need.

6. What are the consequences of poor communication at the end of life?

Poor communication may result in a failure of the clinician to understand what the patient knows about their illness and what they want to know. This can lead to a failure to understand and carry out the patient's preferences. In one study, only 30% of elderly patient's wishes were recorded accurately in their notes (Heyland et al. 2013).

Poor communication risks the patient and family misunderstanding important pieces of information or feeling uninvolved in decision-making (Ahronheim et al. 1996; Royal College of Physicians 2016). Unclear communication is associated with reduced quality of life in cancer patients (Kerr et al. 2003). Inadequate communication can lead to the development of dissatisfaction and distrust for patients and their families (National Audit Office 2008; Neuberger et al. 2013; Royal College of Physicians 2016).

Poor communication causes distress for patients and relatives (Office of National Statistics 2016) including increased risk of depression for bereaved relatives (Wright et al. 2008). Poor communication is one of the biggest causes for unresolved complaints from families about end of life care in UK hospitals (Parliamentary and Health Service Ombudsman 2015) and can be a cause for litigation. Failure to discuss care towards the end of life is more likely to result in aggressive medical treatment which is associated with reduced quality of life for the patients (Wright et al. 2008).

There may be consequences of poor communication for health professionals as well with evidence of negative emotional impact and increased burnout in staff who felt poorly resourced to manage these conversations (Maguire and Pitceathly 2002; Gordon 2003).

7. Guidance around of communicating at the end of life

There have been several protocols developed to support communication of bad news such as SPIKES (Baile et al. 2000) and ABCDE (Rabow and McPhee 1999) which identify the stages to consider when approaching a conversation about end of life care. These are expanded on below, to incorporate all conversations about end of life care, and to move away from the conversation as a single event.

(i) Preparation

It is worth rehearsing the basic rules for good communication which also apply to conversations at the end of life. Firstly, it is important to ensure you have as much information as is available about the patient's medical condition. Partly this is a process of collecting facts, but it also an opportunity to consider where you think the patient is in their illness. Are there markers of advanced disease? Have they been deteriorating recently? Are they at a low level of function due to the progression of their disease? All of these may suggest a shorter prognosis.

It is also an opportunity to review the sort of information that the patient may want to know. If you think about prognosis in advance you will not feel at such a loss when the patient asks you. What do you expect to happen in this disease? For patients who are helped by having information, specific information about how health will change can be very useful. It may be that the view of an expert will be needed if the disease is unusual or one you have not come across before.

If possible, give the patient the opportunity to have someone with them when you start the conversation with them. A relative or friend can provide emotional support during the conversation, and afterwards too. It is helpful for the patient to have someone there to hear the same information, as they may not take in much if they become distressed. The companion can act not only to remember information, but also to clarify anything that was not explained clearly enough. Asking a patient if they wish to bring someone with them can be awkward as it feels as if you are telling them there is "bad news" before you have even started the conversation. When you arrange to speak to the patient you can suggest that their results will be available on such a day or at a certain time and they may wish to have someone with them when you talk. This does require some forethought but planning these conversations will often result in a better experience for both patient and professional.

It is often helpful to have a professional colleague with you when you are planning an end of life conversation. They can support you if the conversation becomes difficult or you dry up, they can write a contemporaneous note of the conversation and they may be able to stay with the patient afterwards to answer questions and offer support. This is particularly important if you are time pressured.

The environment for the conversation also needs to be planned. As much as possible, you should ensure you are in a private area where everyone can be seated. In hospital wards this may be challenging when the patient is bed bound, however drawing curtains or screens around the bed space can at least give the feeling of privacy.

It is very important to try to be on eye level with the patient to increase trust and improve rapport (Rosenzweig 2012). If the patient is lying in bed, then sitting or crouching down next to them can make the biggest difference in putting the patient at ease and reducing the power imbalance that patients often feel when talking to doctors especially. However, be aware that too much eye contact can cause discomfort, just as too little can promote distrust.

(ii) Opening the conversation

Opening conversations about end of life can be challenging. It is difficult to know where to start as we don't know how the patient will react. Therefore, the best place to begin is to find out what the patient understands. The next step is to find out how much information the patient wants. Finally, we need to have strategies for opening the conversation in a way that allows us to stop the conversation at the right time for the patient. Thus, in contrast to the belief and behaviour of many clinicians, good communication around the end of life care involves more listening than talking.

However, some talking is required, and for those less confident in communicating at the end of life, it may be worth rehearsing the words you will use to open the conversation before you begin. In order to establish what the patients knows, use open questions such as "what do you know about your illness?", "what do you understand is going on with your health?" and "what do you think might happen to your health in the future?". Allow the patient the time to consider the question in case they have not done so already. Some patients are tempted to make light of their concerns initially, and you may need to allow time for the conversation to develop rather than trying to push it on too quickly.

(iii) Next steps

The way that the patient responds will guide you to the next step, so active listening is essential. If they deny any problem with their health or any worries about the future, then you know that either they do not understand the seriousness of their condition, or that they know but are choosing to be in denial. Alternatively, the patient may suggest that they understand their health is deteriorating. Either way you now need to explore how much information the patient wishes to have.

This can be asked directly, "are you the sort of person who likes to have all the information about your health, or do you prefer not to know all the details?" You can also approach this by giving the patient a clue that there is more information and waiting for their reply. Asking, "I am quite worried about your health/scan/results" is one way of doing this. You need to wait, possibly in silence whilst the patient absorbs this and considers how they want to respond. Possibly the biggest mistake health professionals make is to try to fill silences by talking, when waiting a few minutes will allow the patient to tell them exactly what they know and want to know (Maguire and Pitceathly 2002).

If the patient suggests that they want to hear more, you are then able to take the conversation on a stage further. It is still best not to make assumptions that they want all the information you might have to give in one go. Instead proceed with small chunks of information after which you pause and allow the patient time to reflect and respond. Expressing your concern about the situation can help the patients understanding. Warning shots as you go along gives the patient the opportunity to go at their speed and to stop when they have heard as much as they can cope with at that time. Examples of these would be, "we think it could be serious" or "we are not sure we can make you better".

Use language that can be easily understood by the patient. Try to imagine you are explaining something to one of your family. Avoid using any jargon or medical abbreviations. The words you use should also match the words the patient uses as much as possible. If the patient prefers to describe their problem as a "weak heart" or a "lung tumour" it is helpful if you reflect this way of describing their problem rather than "heart failure" or "lung cancer".

(iv) Go at the patient's pace

It is important to individualise each conversation and to try to make it about the patient and what they need, rather than about a transfer of information. As health professionals with information to share or information to find out, we arrive at these conversations with our own agendas. It is helpful to be aware of your agenda and to be ready to adjust your approach based on what the patient needs. Some patients will want you to be very direct and you may have to adjust your sensitive approach and be blunter than you would choose to be. For other patients, you will leave the first conversation without understanding everything you wish to or saying everything you know. Because of this, end of life communications should be thought about as a process and not as an event (Chapple et al. 2011). This contrasts with the notion of "breaking bad news" which suggests a single conversation.

(v) Listening and responding to cues

Patients reveal cues and concerns during conversations that are intended to give us information about what they think or feel (Zimmermann and Del Piccolo 2007). Improving your ability to pick up and respond to these clues can improve the quality of your communication and the amount of significant information the patient discloses in return (Maguire et al. 1996). Picking up and responding appropriately to cues has also been shown to shorten the consultation time (Levinson, Horawara-Bhat and Lamb 2000). However, clinicians tend to miss or ignore cues (Butow et al. 2002), or respond in inappropriate ways by interrupting, discouraging discussion or by giving advice (Fallowfield et al. 2002; Zimmermann and Del Piccolo 2007). Specific training can improve recognition of, and appropriate response to, communication cues from patients (Moore et al. 2013; Fallowfield et al. 2002).

Cues can be verbal or non-verbal. Verbal cues can be explicit such as "I need you tell me directly what is happening" or "I don't want to hear this". Sometimes it is too difficult for a patient to say they don't want to continue a conversation. In this case they may use other cues which you need to look out for such as changing the subject or more subtle messages such as, "I'm rather tired, can we talk some other time?"

Non-verbal cues are usually described as those expressed through posture or body movement (Zimmermann and Del Piccolo 2007). They may be very clear, such as a patient closing their eyes, crying, turning their face or body away, or they may be more difficult to interpret, for instance, the patient avoids eye contact or goes quiet. It is important to recognise and acknowledge that the patient is feeling something, even if you don't know what it is. "I think you are finding this difficult....?", would be one way of doing this which allows the patient to explain if they wish to. Expressions of empathy are appropriate when a patient is emotionally affected by the conversation – this is a human and humane response. Clinician expressions of empathy also increase the likelihood that the patient will make significant disclosures (Maguire et al. 1996).

(vi) Using silences and avoiding blocking statements

Silences can be helpful or awkward and as such require a clinician more confident in communicating to avoid a negative impact. Silence can be an opportunity for the patient to reflect and respond – a so called invitational silence, which often precedes important disclosures on the part of the patient (Eide et al. 2004). This is also an opportunity for the professional to pause and watch for clues about how the patient feels (Back et al. 2009).

Experience in communication also helps clinicians to avoid using responses which can block further disclosure from the patient. These responses include offering premature reassurances, downplaying the emotion expressed by the patient, playing down the issues changing the subject or using humour inappropriately (Maguire and Pitceathly 2002). These behaviours are often a consequence of discomfort on the part of the clinician from a reluctance to engage further in an uncomfortable conversation.

(vii) Dealing with strong emotions

Conversations at the end of life can raise strong emotions in patients and their families. This can be a source of concern for those leading the communication and is a barrier for some to starting the conversation at all. Anxiety, sadness, shock, and anger/frustration are all common occurring in up to 70% of end of life conversations (Alexander et al. 2014). The expressions of these emotions can leave professionals feeling at a loss for how to respond. They may struggle to know what to say to make the patient feel better. It is important not to ignore these expressions of emotion but to be empathic. Compassionate responses to emotional expressions during difficult conversations can reduce patient anxiety a year later (Schofield et al. 2003).

(viii) Uncertainty and hope

Uncertainty about the future for a patient can prevent healthcare professionals starting a conversation about end of life care (Brighton and Bristowe 2016). It is difficult to embark on a conversation when there is so much unknown including prognosis and what the patient's deteriorating health will look like. In addition, we may be concerned about the negative impact on the patient of having hope crushed (Lakin and Jacobsen 2019). Some patients and their families reject information about the future which is entirely negative, preferring to focus on optimism (Koenig and Gates-Williams 1995). Clinicians may feel they need to choose to present one option – that of preserving hope or of encouraging patients and families to prepare for death (Back, Arnold and Quill 2003). A more successful strategy may be to acknowledge the uncertainty but present possibilities for the future which encompass both our hopeful and pessimistic views of the future (Lakin and Jacobsen 2019). This "hope for the best but prepare for the worst" approach (Kahana et al. 2011; Back et al. 2003), can be helpful for clinicians, patients and their families.

(ix) Ending the conversation and considerations afterwards

How we close conversations about end of life care is important in terms of choosing the right place in the conversation, checking understanding and planning for further discussions (Baile et al. 2000; Rabow and McPhee 1999). The conversation should stop when the patient has had the right amount of discussion for them. This will vary enormously between patients and requires the clinician to be sufficiently skilled not to push the discussion further than the patient is ready for.

If significant information has been discussed it is helpful to check the patient and family's understanding (Baile et al. 2000). Significant discrepancies in understanding can be revealed by this process which can then be corrected (Quirt et al. 1997). If a discussion has been distressing, it is useful to bring the conversation onto less emotional subjects so that the patient and family are not so distressed when they leave. A follow up discussion can also be offered to the patient to address any questions and continue the conversation if desired.

After the conversation, it is important to think about how the health professionals are feeling, especially if the discussion has been difficult or involved strong expressions of emotion from patient or family. Even when experienced physicians follow appropriate communicating strategies, they can be left with distress from the encounter which is long lasting, even if the patient's distress as well managed (Ptacek et al. 1999).

8. Managing conflict in end of life communication

Conflict can arise for a variety of different reasons in end of life care conversations including loss of trust in healthcare professionals, reluctance to accept new information, inconsistent or confusing messages from the healthcare team, unrealistic expectations, different cultural approaches to communication and different cultural or spiritual beliefs. Skilled communication is the most powerful tool to reducing and resolving the conflict. Too often, however, the aim of the communication is to persuade and cajole, where a more effective approach would be to reach a consensus by compromise on both sides.

Firstly, use of the type of communication skills described in this chapter can maintain trust of patients and relatives and avoid conflict arising. Being alert to the possibility of these conversations causing distress and disagreement may help us to avoid some conflict, or to recognise tensions arising at an early stage.

Once conflict is recognised it is helpful to arrange a meeting with the patient and/or family members to discuss the situation. The purpose of this meeting is not primarily to encourage the patient and family to accept your point of view, but to build trust and a common understanding of the situation. This may take more than a single discussion and this process cannot be rushed. This may be frustrating when, for instance, a patient is dying, and the healthcare team feel continued treatment is causing distress for no benefit. However, the alternative is that both the family and healthcare team become more fixed in their opposing positions and more inflexible as time goes on. This can result in total breakdown of communication and trust between the health care team and family, with disastrous results.

Clarify what the patient and family understand and what they think will happen in the future. This may expose reasons for the conflict and suggest how it may be addressed. For instance, the family may describe previous events where they lost trust in healthcare systems which have influenced their approach to this situation. If the disagreement is based on misunderstandings, then appropriate explanation may help the family understand your different perspectives. Be aware that there may also be some reluctance to accept a pessimistic prognosis, because of the distress this causes, or because of a religious belief that dictates that only God can decide what happens in the future. The use of the "hope for the best but prepare for the worst" approach is very useful here.

Involving others such as clinical ethicists, palliative care specialists or chaplains in end of life family conferences can reduce conflict (Schneiderman et al. 2003; Curtis et al. 2001). Second opinions can also be helpful to reassure the family, and an early offer of a second opinion can reflect your willingness to review your decision which may in itself help to rebuild trust.

In situations where the patient is unable or unwilling to be involved in communication, we need to involve families to find out what the patient would want us to do. When families are involved the clinicians have a better idea of the patients' preferences, although a minority of family members act against the wishes of the patient (Hauke et al. 2011).

Acknowledge the uncertainty of the situation and the fact that the family know the patient much better than you do. Express your desire for the best outcome for the patient, just as the family do. Identify and empathise with the emotions that the patient and family are experiencing. Expressing your feelings of compassion may help to build trust. It also helps to focus the patient and family on their emotion rather than on resisting what they see as your agenda. Offering the involvement of a palliative care team to provide symptom control and emotional support can reinforce your expressed desire to help.

9.2 Conclusion

Communication around the end of life can be challenging because discussing the possibility that someone may die can give rise to strong emotions. Globally there are different expectations about truth telling and sharing of bad news. It is crucial for healthcare professionals to be aware of the cultural norms of the patient and their family to avoid distress and unnecessary conflict. Conflict can also be limited by skilled communication that focuses on listening. Maintaining trust with the patient and family is important to enable any sort of therapeutic relationship to continue. Second opinions can be useful for both healthcare professionals and patients and families. Finally it is vital that staff have support to manage the emotional impact of these conversations on themselves.

References

Ahronheim, J., R. Morrison, S. Baskin, J. Morris, and D. Meier. 1996. Treatment of the dying in the acute care hospital. *Archives of Internal Medicine* 156: 2094–2100.

Alexander, S., S. Ladwig, S. Norton, D. Gramling, J. Davis, M. Metzger, J. DeLuca, and R. Gramling. 2014. Emotional distress and compassionate responses in palliative care decision-making consultations. *Journal of Palliative Medicine* 17 (5): 579–584.

Almack, K., K. Cox, N. Moghaddam, K. Pollock, and J. Seymour. 2012. After you: Conversations between patients and healthcare professionals in planning for end of life care. *BMC Palliative Care* 11: 15.

Back, A., R. Arnold, and T. Quill. 2003. Hope for the best, and prepare for the worst. *Annals of Internal Medicine* 138 (5): 439–443.

Back, A., S. Bauer-Wu, C. Rushton, and J. Halifax. 2009. Compassionate silence in the patient–clinician encounter: A contemplative approach. *Journal of Palliative Medicine* 12 (12): 1113–1117.

Baile, W., R. Buckman, R. Lenzi, G. Glober, E. Beale, and A. Kudelka. 2000. SPIKES—A six-step protocol for delivering bad news: Application to the patient with cancer. *The Oncologist* 5 (4): 302–311.

Barclay, S., and J. Maher. 2010. Having the difficult conversations about the end of life. *BMJ* 341: 653–655.

Blackhall, L., S. Murphy, G. Frank, V. Michel, and S. Azen. 1995. Ethnicity and attitudes toward patient autonomy. *Journal of the American Medical Association* 274 (10): 820–825.

Brighton, L., and K. Bristowe. 2016. Communication in palliative care: Talking about the end of life, before the end of life. *Postgraduate Medical Journal* 92: 466–470.

Butow, P., R. Brown, S. Cogar, M. Tattersall, and S. Dunn. 2002. Oncologists' reactions to cancer patients' verbal cues. *Psycho-Oncology* 11 (1): 47–58.

Chapple, A., J. Evans, A. McPherson, and S. Payne. 2011. Patients with pancreatic cancer and relatives talk about preferred place of death and what influenced their preferences: A qualitative study. *BMJ Support Palliative Care* 1 (3): 291–295.

Crawley, L., P. Marshall, B. Lo, and B. Koenig. 2002. Strategies for culturally effective end-of-life care. *Annals of Internal Medicine* 136 (9): 673–679.

Curtis, J., D. Patrick, S. Shannon, P. Treece, R. Engelberg, and G. Rubenfeld. 2001. The family conference as a focus to improve communication about end-of-life care in the intensive care unit: Opportunities for improvement. *Critical Care Medicine* 29 (Suppl 2): N26–N33.

Davison, S., and C. Simpson. 2006. Hope and advance care planning in patients with end stage renal disease. *BMJ* 333 (7574): 886–890.

Eide, H., V. Quera, P. Graugaard, and A. Finset. 2004. Physician-patient dialogue surrounding patients'expression of concern: Applying sequence analysis to RIAS. *Social Science & Medicine* 59 (1): 145–155.

Eliott, J., and I. Olver. 2009. Hope, life and death: A qualitative analysis of dying cancer patients' talk about hope. *Death Studies* 33: 609–638.

Fallowfield, L., V. Jenkins, F. Farewell, J. Saul, A. Duffy, and R. Eves. 2002. Efficacy of a cancer research UK communication skills training model for oncologists: A randomized trial. *The Lancet* 359: 650–656.

Fawole, O., S. Dy, R. Wilson, B. Lau, K. Martinez, C. Apostol, D. Vollenweider, E. Bass, and R. Aslakson. 2013. A systematic review of communication quality improvement interventions for patients with advanced and serious illness. *Journal of General Internal Medicine* 28 (4): 570–577.

Gordon, G. 2003. Care not cure: Dialogues at the transition. *Patient Education and Counseling* 50 (1): 95–98.

Haidet, P., M. Hamel, R. Davis, N. Wenger, D. Reding, P. Kussin, A. Connors, J. Lynn, J. Weeks, and R. Phillips. 1998. Outcomes, preferences for resuscitation, and physician-patient communication among patients with metastatic colorectal cancer. SUPPORT Investigators. Study to Understand Prognoses and Preferences for Outcomes and Risks of Treatments. *The American Journal of Medicine* 105 (3): 222–229.

Hauke, D., S. Reiter-Theil, E. Hoster, W. Hiddemann, and E. Winkler. 2011. The role of relatives in decisions concerning life-prolonging treatment inpatients with end-stage malignant disorders: Informants, advocates or surrogate decision-makers. *Annals of Oncology* 22: 2667–2674.

Heyland, D., D. Barwich, D. Pichora, P. Dodek, F. Lamontagne, J. You, C. Tayler, P. Porterfield, T. Sinuff, J. Simon, and for the ACCEPT (Advance Care Planning Evaluation in Elderly Patients) Study Team and the Canadian Researchers at the End of Life Network (CARENET). 2013. Failure to engage hospitalized elderly patients and their families in advance care planning. *JAMA Internal Medicine* 173 (9): 778–787.

Hoffmann, T., and C. Del Mar. 2015. Patients' expectations of the benefits and harms of treatments, screening, and tests: A systematic review. *JAMA Internal Medicine* 175 (2): 274–286.

Hsieh, J.G., and Y.W. Wang. 2012. Application of signs of dying identified in traditional Chinese, Tibetan, and modern Western medicine in terminal care. *The Tzu Chi Medical Journal* 24 (1): 12–15. https://doi.org/10.1016/j.tcmj.2012.02.004.

Hunt, L. 1998. Moral reasoning and the meaning of cancer: Causal explanations of oncologists and patients in southern Mexico. *Medical Anthropology Quarterly* 12: 298–318.

Kahana, B., E. Kahana, L. Lovegreen, and J. Brown. 2011. Hoping for the best and preparing for the worst: End-of-life attitudes of the elderly. *BMJ Supportive & Palliative Care* 1: 93.

Kerr, J., J. Engel, A. Schlesinger-Raab, H. Sauer, and D. Holzel. 2003. Doctor-patient communication. *Diseases of the Colon and Rectum* 46 (8): 1038–1046.

Koenig, B., and J. Gates-Williams. 1995. Understanding cultural difference in caring for dying patients. *The Western Journal of Medicine* 163: 244–249.

Lakin, J., and J. Jacobsen. 2019. Softening our approach to discussing prognosis. *JAMA Internal Medicine* 179 (1): 5–6.

Levinson, W., R. Horawara-Bhat, and J. Lamb. 2000. A study of patient clues and physician responses in primary care and surgical settings. *Journal of the American Medical Association* 284: 1021–1027.

Maguire, P., and C. Pitceathly. 2002. Key communication skills and how to acquire them. *BMJ* 325: 697–700. https://doi.org/10.1136/bmj.325.7366.697.

Maguire, P., A. Faulkner, K. Booth, C. Elliot, and V. Hillier. 1996. Helping cancer patients disclose their concerns. *European Journal of Cancer* 32: 78–81.

Moore, P., S. Rivera Mercado, M. Grez Artigues, and T. Lawrie. 2013. Communication skills training for healthcare professionals working with people who have cancer. *Cochrane Database of Systematic Reviews* 7 (3): CD003751.

National Audit Office. 2008. *Patient and Carer experiences regarding end of life Care in England*. London: National Audit Office. Available at; https://www.nao.org.uk/wp-content/uploads/2008/11/07081043_patientcarersurvey.pdf. Accessed 11Jan 2019.

Neuberger, J., C. Guthrie, D. Aaronovitch, K. Hameed, T. Bonser, R. Harris, E. Jackson, and S. Waller. 2013. *More care, less pathway: A review of the Liverpool care pathway*. London: Department of Health. Available at: https://assets.publishing.service.gov.uk/government/

uploads/system/uploads/attachment_data/file/212450/Liverpool_Care_Pathway.pdf. Accessed 15 Mar 2019.
Office for National Statistics, NHS England. 2016. *National Survey of Bereaved People, 2014*. [Data collection]. UK Data Service. SN: 7978. Available at https://doi.org/10.5255/UKDA-SN-7978-1. Accessed 20 Feb 2019.
Parliamentary and Health Service Ombudsman. 2015. *Dying without dignity: Investigations by the parliamentary and health service ombudsman into complaints about end of life care*. https://www.ombudsman.org.uk/sites/default/files/Dying_without_dignity.pdf. Accessed 16 Mar 2019.
Periyakoil, V., E. Neri, and H. Kraemer. 2015. No easy talk: A mixed-methods study of doctor reported barriers to conducting effective end-of-life conversations with diverse patients. *PLoS One* 10 (4): e0122321.
Ptacek, J., E. Fries, T. Eberhardt, and J. Ptacek. 1999. Breaking bad news to patients; Physicians' perceptions of the process. *Support Care Cancer* 7: 113–120.
Quirt, C., W. McKillop, A. Ginsberg, L. Sheldon, M. Brundage, P. Dixon, and L. Ginsburg. 1997. Do doctors know when their patients don't? A survey of doctor-patient communication in lung cancer. *Lung Cancer* 18 (1): 1–20.
Rabow, M., and S. McPhee. 1999. Beyond breaking bad news: How to help patients who suffer. *The Western Journal of Medicine* 171 (4): 260–263.
Rosenberg, A.R., H. Starks, Y. Unguru, C. Feudtner, and D. Diekema. 2017. Truth telling in the setting of cultural differences and incurable pediatric illness: A review. *JAMA Pediatrics* 171 (11): 1113–1119. https://doi.org/10.1001/jamapediatrics.2017.2568.
Rosenzweig, M. 2012. Breaking bad news: A guide for effective and empathetic communication. *The Nurse Practitioner* 37 (2): 1–4.
Royal College of Physicians. 2016. *End of life care audit – Dying in hospital*. London: RCP. Available at https://www.rcplondon.ac.uk/projects/outputs/end-life-care-audit-dying-hospital-national-report-england-2016. Accessed 13 Feb 2019.
Scheidt, Carl Eduard, Alexander Wunsch, Hamid Afshar, Farzad Goli, Azadeh Malekian, Mohammad Reza Sharbafchi, Masoud Ferdosi, Mitra Molaeinezhad, and Farzad Taslimi. 2017. Breaking bad news: Different approaches in different countries of Iran and Germany-an expert panel. *International Journal of Body, Mind and Culture* 4: 108–114.
Schneiderman, L., T. Gilmer, H. Teetzel, D. Dugan, J. Blustein, R. Cranford, K. Briggs, G. Komatsu, P. Goodman-Crews, F. Cohn, and E. Young. 2003. Effect of ethics consultations on nonbeneficial life-sustaining treatments in the intensive care setting: A randomised controlled trial. *The Journal of the American Medical Association* 290: 1166–1172.
Schofield, P., P. Butow, J. Thompson, M. Tattersall, L. Beeney, and S. Dunn. 2003. Psychological responses of patients receiving a diagnosis of cancer. *Annals of Oncology* 14 (1): 48–56.
Stewart, M.A. 1995. Effective physician-patient communication and health outcomes: A review. *Canadian Medical Association Journal* 152: 1423–1433.
Stewart, A., J. Teno, D. Patrick, and J. Lynne. 1999. The concept of quality of life of dying persons in the context of health care. *Journal of Pain and Symptom Management* 17 (2): 93–108.
SUPPORT Principal Investigators. (1995) A controlled trial to improve care for seriously ill hospitalized patients. The Study to Understand Prognoses and Preferences for Outcomes and Risks of Treatments (SUPPORT). [published erratum appears in *JAMA* 1996 Apr 24; 275(16):1232]. *JAMA* 274(20):1591–1598.
Teno, J., R. Hakim, W. Knaus, N. Wenger, R. Phillips, A. Wu, P. Layde, A. Connors Jr., N. Dawson, J. Lynn, and the SUPPORT investigators. 1995. Preferences for cardiopulmonary resuscitation: Physician-patient agreement and hospital resource use. The SUPPORT investigators. *The Journal of General Internal Medicine, 1995* 10 (4): 179–186.
Teno, J., V. Casey, L. Welch, and S. Edgman-Levitan. 2001. Patient focused, family centered end-of-life medical care: Views of the guidelines and bereaved family members. *Journal of Pain and Symptom Management* 22 (3): 738–751.

Wright, A., B. Zhang, A. Ray, J. Mack, E. Trice, T. Balboni, S. Mitchell, V. Jackson, S. Block, P. Maciejewski, H. Prigerson, et al. 2008. Associations between end-of-life discussions, patient mental health, medical care near death, and caregiver bereavement adjustment. *Journal of the American Medical Association* 300: 1665–1673.

Zhang, A., and L. Siminoff. 2003. Silence and cancer: Why do families and patients fail to communicate? *Health Communication* 15 (4): 415–429.

Zimmermann, C., and L. Del Piccolo. 2007. Cues and concerns by patients in medical consultations: A literature review. *Psycholo Review* 133 (3): 438–463.

Part III
Medico-Legal Proposals

Chapter 10
Advance Care Planning

Paul Paes

Abstract This chapter discusses the important issue of Advance Care Planning as a means of enabling people to understand what is happening to them in the face of a terminal illness, and give them the opportunity to regain some control over events. It describes what Advance Care Planning is, and the process that takes place. It highlights current barriers to the process and the potential outputs that may emerge in the form of different tools. Some of the ethical issues involved in Advance Care Planning are discussed, particularly around who has the power to make decisions, what is allowed legally, the ideas of net benefit and "ordinary" versus "extraordinary treatments, as well as mental capacity. The effectiveness of Advance Care Planning is considered, before reflecting on the core element of this process- good, honest communication which enables people to think realistically about the future.

Keywords Planning · Advance · Communication · Ethics · Autonomy

A key skill of being a health professional is to recognise a change in someone's condition and intervene to address the new situation. Good health care is anticipating the change before it happens and planning the intervention before it is needed. That is the essence of Advance Care Planning- anticipating a change and planning for it.

In end of life care, a patient's health is deteriorating. Palliative care is about intervening to try to maintain quality of life and improve the situation for patients and their family, even if the underlying diagnosis cannot be treated. As with other health problems, good palliative care is about anticipating and planning the intervention before it is needed. Thus, a key reason to identify that a patient is reaching the end of their life is that it allows us to plan ahead and to offer care that meets the wishes and needs of patients. This gives patients, families and health professionals some basis on which to navigate the final stages of illness, albeit through a period which

P. Paes (✉)
Newcastle University, Newcastle upon Tyne, UK
e-mail: Paul.Paes@newcastle.ac.uk

P. Mallia et al. (eds.), *Challenges to the Global Issue of End of Life Care*, Advancing Global Bioethics 17, https://doi.org/10.1007/978-3-030-86386-9_10

still contains uncertainty. Crucially it allows people to exercise a degree of control over their lives at a time when everything may seem to be spiralling out of control.

This chapter will explore what Advance Care Planning is, focus on how it is practised and address some of the cultural, legal and ethical issues that arise from the process.

10.1 What Is Advance Care Planning?

Advance Care Planning (ACP) is the process of:

1. Thinking about
2. Discussing and
3. Making plans for the future

It is done in anticipation of something adverse happening and in anticipation of the potential for the patient to lose the capacity to be involved in making a decision. For an individual, ACP can involve all three aspects or they may find it useful to think and/or talk without making a concrete plan. The thinking and discussing aspects of ACP may be as useful as any plan that emerges.

Addressing current problems should always be a priority in end of life care, but perhaps greater skill is required by the healthcare team when attempting to anticipate and plan for future problems. Decision making in this situation takes a number of forms and must comply with the legal and ethical frameworks of individual countries. These outputs may take the form of patient-driven tools for example wills, powers of attorney and advance directives; or professionally driven tools e.g. Do Not Attempt Resuscitation (DNAR) forms or Treatment Escalation Plans. Whatever the output of ACP, the starting point is a conversation, or thoughts and reflections on their current and future situation.

10.2 Advance Care Planning Conversations

There are a number of challenges in ACP discussions. Thinking about the future can only happen if people have a realistic understanding of the present. That may not always be the case as some patients have a sub-optimal level of discussion with their health professionals about their condition, despite a desire for more information and involvement in current decision-making processes. This means they have limited discussions about the future with their health professionals and find it hard to raise issues (MacPherson et al. 2013).

There are some paradoxes to overcome in talking about the future: often, professionals wait for patients to approach them to discuss end of life issues, while patients wait for health professionals to raise the topic and, it seems, want their health professionals to open up the discussion (Heffner et al. 2000). This lack of dialogue can leave patients uncertain about their future and prognosis, thereby being unable to effectively plan for either. Moreover, patients often adapt to living with a terminal illness by dealing with it on a day to day basis, and not by thinking ahead (MacPherson et al. 2013). These factors means that conversations between patients and their families about the future and their wishes are limited (Churm 2016) perhaps underpinned by misunderstanding or uncertainty.

Effective planning cannot take place without people being fully informed in the first place. Engagement with ACP is associated with people who have a better understanding of their illness (Wagner et al. 2010). A particular challenge to society is that engagement is associated with a higher level of education (Wagner et al. 2010), white populations and older people (Reynolds et al. 2008) though most research on ACP has taken place in western populations.

Nevertheless, while there are significant obstacles, discussions about ACP are important because they increase patient satisfaction (Detering et al. 2010) and positively affect anxiety and depression (Pautex et al. 2008). They also allow patients to open up and prompt further discussion about future care with their relatives (Smucker et al. 1993).

Opening up a dialogue about the present and future need not be complicated. Some simple, open ended, questions will usually allow a conversation to commence. These include:

- What is your understanding about …?
- What have you been told about …?
- What do you expect to happen?
- What are your priorities now and in the future?
- How would you like…?
- Have you spoken to your family about …?

These are simple questions to ask but can open up a range of areas for discussion. That can sometimes cause anxiety in health professionals, who may not feel confident to deal with the responses, questions or emotions that may then emerge. Training in this area is important, either face to face or on-line using large scale e-learning programmes for example, the e-learning End of Life Care for All programme (E-ELCA 2010), but should not be an excuse for avoiding straightforward human conversations which need not be over-medicalised.

A systematic review showed that when patients and families are asked what is important to them at the end of their life, the importance of communication shines through, even in those areas that are not overtly called "communication" (Virdun et al. 2015) (Table 10.1).

Involvement in decision making is also highly valued. A study asked patients and non-professional carers to rank the importance of key factors linked to a good death for patients and their carers (Davies et al. 2016) (Fig. 10.1).

These studies help to inform the sorts of areas that might be included in discussions about future care, as well as highlighting subtly different priorities for patients and their families/carers. Areas are considered important to think about in an ACP discussion include:

Table 10.1 Most important factors at the end of life (Virdun et al. 2015)

	Patient	Family
1	Effective Communication and shared decision making	Expert care
2	Expert care	Effective Communication and shared decision making
3	Respectful and compassionate care	Respectful and compassionate care
4	Trust and confidence in clinicians	Trust and confidence in clinicians
5	Adequate environment for care Minimising burden	Financial affairs

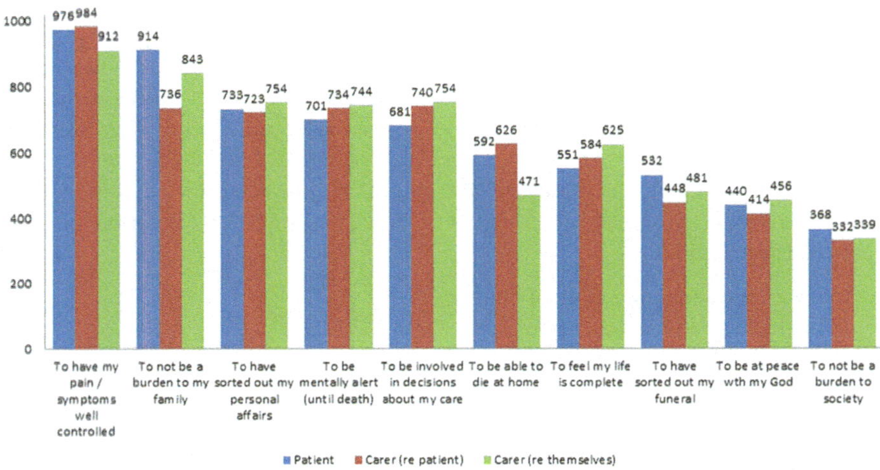

Fig. 10.1 Key factors linked to a good death. (Davies et al. 2016)

- The amount of information they would like to have about their condition as it changes, and how they would like to be informed
- The level of involvement they would like in on-going decision making
- General care preferences
- Financial and legal issues
- Their preferences over how and where they are cared for as their condition changes
- Their preferences over how and where they are cared for in the last days of their life
- Management of deteriorations or complications of their illness, including levels of escalation
- Aspects of nutrition and hydration
- Aspects of personal care such as continence
- Organ donation

Perhaps the most important aspect is to cover any areas that patients want to bring up. Sometimes giving people information or resources about Advance Care Planning can act as a useful prompt, but should not be a substitute for a conversation.

10.3 Outputs of ACP

When a patient's condition deteriorates the loss of control they experience can be overwhelming. Involving them in decision making restores some control over events. Literature in this area suggests that patients seldom get the chance to have these discussions before emergency situations arise and, furthermore, that such discussions would be welcome (Goodridge 2006). There is limited awareness of the ACP process in many patients especially those with chronic problems (Churm 2016). ACP is a voluntary process. That process may simply be awareness and thinking about the future; it may lead to conversations between patients, families and health professionals or it may ultimately lead to specific formal outputs or plans. There is currently a low conversion from ACP discussions to the development of an actual plan though that increases if discussions take place with a skilled professional (Detering et al. 2010).

It is important to recognise that Advance Care Planning decisions only apply if and when a patient loses capacity. Furthermore, a loss of capacity may be transient such as a sudden change in their health status. Patients should be given every chance to regain capacity if a decision can be delayed. Loss of mental capacity often occurs in the last days of life as patients become unconscious. While a patient has capacity they should always be consulted about decision making. Equally patients have the right to, and do change their minds; care should be taken when interpreting plans, and care should be taken to ensure they are evolving plans that are regularly updated.

The outputs of an ACP process vary significantly across the world depending on the legal framework that is in place around mental capacity and anticipatory decision making. This section considers the broad options available but each needs to be interpreted according to individual legislation and guidance applicable in each country.

10.3.1 Patient-Driven Decision Making

There are some simple everyday decisions such as taking out insurance or making a will that can be considered outputs of ACP. They are put in place in order to address a future potential issue or ensure that someone's wishes are carried out. People are more likely to engage in these sorts of practical ACP, which have a clear impact on those who are important to them (Churm 2016). Often these types of decisions are enhanced by being done in collaboration with the expertise of financial or legal advisors. Similarly, while people can make decisions about their health and care on their own, doing it in partnership with health professionals is likely to lead to wiser decision making.

As noted, some patients will be happy simply to discuss what is likely to happen, think about the future and their choices, but not wish to do anything more. There are valid reasons for this (MacPherson et al. 2013):

- they may have a reasonable idea of preferences but not strong enough to want to make future decisions
- they may be unsure how they would feel in the future and may change their mind
- they may wonder whether if they are so ill, whether it would really matter to them what decisions were taken
- People are wary about making decisions for the future when the disease follows an unpredictable course and wonder what the benefit is in any binding decisions
- Choices may be limited if they are very ill so making anticipatory decisions may be pointless because it would not change anything

Additionally, rather than requiring active Shared Decision Making, end-of-life care may 'fall into place' as patients deteriorate without the need for significant forward planning (Drought and Koenig 2002). Other people will prefer to take more control of this process by recording some of their preferences in the form of an ACP document, Advance Statement or other such document. This is a statement reflecting an individual's preferences and aspirations. It can help health professionals identify how the person would like to be treated and record past, present and future wishes. It is the documented result of an ACP discussion. Crucially it is not legally binding, which means that health care professionals need to use their judgement in applying the values/priorities expressed in the document to their decision making. For patients, this aspect addresses a fear that they may commit themselves to a decision which they may later regret. A powerful aspect of an Advance Statement is that it enables views to be communicated, checked, clarified and then shared with others, in particular their family. That has practical benefits, as well as opening up important conversations. A concern is that significant numbers of people are making plans without discussing them with their family (Lamont and Siegler 2000) which may lead to disagreement when it comes to interpreting any plan. More importantly it is a missed opportunity to open up conversations among family members.

As well as setting out advisory preferences, in most countries there are also legally binding options for patients. These include:

- Appointing someone to make decisions on your behalf should you be unable to make those decisions in the future. In the UK and other countries, this is a Lasting Power of Attorney, with a full legal framework setting out the scope and safeguards around such a role. These positions often focus on health and care issues, additionally they can address matters to do with finance and property.

- Living wills, Advance Directives or an Advance Decision to Refuse Treatment (ADRT). This is a decision to refuse specific treatments and, if set out correctly, is a legally binding document. Common treatments that may be refused include resuscitation, ventilation, feeding tubes, intravenous fluids, and antibiotics. The main purpose of these decisions is to avoid prolonging the life, or the dying phase of life in people who wish to allow natural death. In most countries, there is a legal right to refuse treatments but not a legal right to demand treatments. These decisions are closely regulated, being required to set out the particular future circumstances of the anticipated treatment, a clear understanding of the consequences, no signs of coercion, as well as there being nothing to suggest a change in mind between writing the treatment refusal and now. Written Advance Directives are associated with less use of life sustaining treatment and less hospitalisation so can be effective in the right circumstances (Teno et al. 2007; Robinson et al. 2011)

10.3.2 Professionally Driven Decision Making

ACP is a voluntary process that is dependent on patients wishing to plan for anticipated changes in their condition. Whether that takes place or not, healthcare professionals need to have clear management plans, which anticipate and address potential problems. In the vast majority of cases, this should be done with the full involvement of patients unless doing so would cause considerable distress or the patient has lost capacity (in which case there may be a national legal framework to follow).

10.3.3 Clinical Management/Care Plans

The most straightforward option is to simply have a management plan agreed between the health team and the patient to address some of the following:

- What are the most likely clinical problems? Often these will be about exacerbations of an underlying condition, symptoms such as pain and potential acute events such as infections or thrombo-embolic disease.
- What is the best management of these problems? What clinical signs should people look out for? What treatment would work for this individual patient? What is the appropriate escalation/ceiling of care? What can be managed at home and when should an admission to hospital be considered?

In some areas, a number of specific tools are used to aid and document this process, varying between countries:

10.3.4 Do Not Attempt Cardio-Pulmonary Resuscitation (DNACPR) Documents

These are documented decisions about how a cardio-pulmonary arrest should be managed. A DNACPR decision means that no attempt will be made to resuscitate a patient if they have a cardiac arrest. This may be appropriate in a number of circumstances towards the end of life. They are usually advisory decisions to guide a clinician faced with managing this situation; to make it legally binding would require a form of Advance Directive. This is discussed further from an ethical perspective.

10.3.5 Emergency Healthcare Plans

These documents are designed to give a specific plan to address an anticipated clinical problem where the right treatment is required promptly. Such a form is used as part of the Deciding Right initiative, a programme designed to encourage discussion and future planning (NHS North East 2011). These plans are very specific to individual situations and may cover a particular treatment, for example how to manage seizures in someone who is no longer able to manage tablets. They follow a logical process of planning:

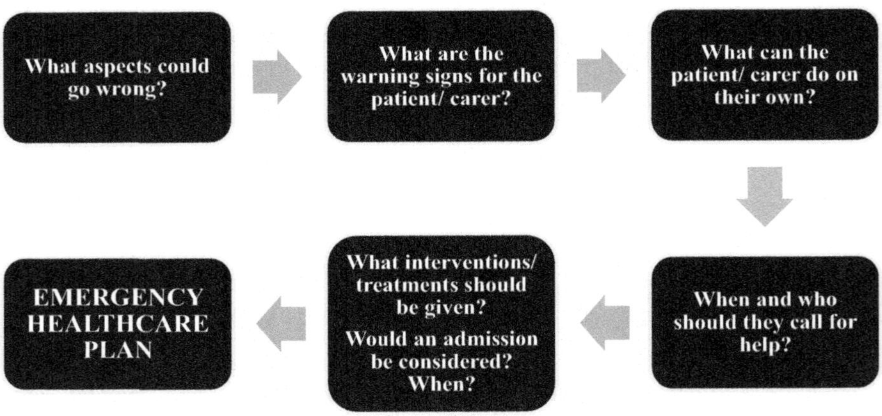

10.3.6 Treatment Escalation Plans (TEPs)

TEPs are growing in popularity, designed to be used for patients who are deteriorating and for whom acute problems are anticipated (Paes and O'Neill 2012). As a patient's health deteriorates, their ability to benefit from specific treatments lessens. Treatment escalation planning looks at specific treatments and considers whether a patient is likely to benefit. Importantly this needs to be an evolving document as a patient's situation changes. It allows both quick escalations of care where that will make a difference (sometimes patients considered "palliative" are undertreated) as well as ruling out treatments that are no longer effective or desired (sometimes patients considered "palliative" are subjected to burdensome treatments with little chance of success). The type of decisions included in a TEP can be seen below, based on an individual's World Health Organisation performance status, and therefore their ability to benefit from a treatment:

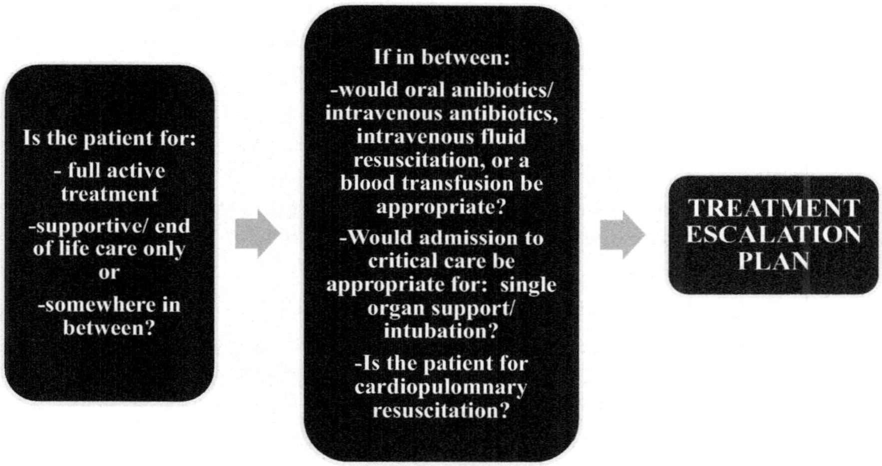

An Emergency Healthcare Plan is likely to be useful in managing a specific anticipated problem with a specific treatment plan. A Treatment Escalation Plan may be more helpful where a number of potential problems may arise, and guidance is required as to which specific treatments may be of benefit to a patient. Importantly clinical management plans, Emergency Healthcare Plans and Treatment Escalation Plans are advisory plans and should guide clinical assessment and judgement, rather than replacing it. Increasingly processes are evolving which try to bring some of these processes and documents together (Fritz et al. 2017). All of these approaches should include patients where possible in joint decision making and be consistent with any ACP discussions.

10.4 ACP- an International Perspective

ACP has been evolving over time, resulting in wide variation in what it means and how it is practised. The European Association for Palliative Care (EAPC) attempted to reach a common understanding by setting up an international taskforce from eight countries to carry out a Delphi exercise among 109 experts, the vast majority

(82) from Europe with the rest from North America and Australia (Rietjens et al. 2017). They sought to define Advance Care Planning:

> Advance care planning enables individuals who have decisional capacity to identify their values, to reflect upon the meanings and consequences of serious illness scenarios, to define goals and preferences for future medical treatment and care, and to discuss these with family and healthcare providers. ACP addresses individuals' concerns across the physical, psychological, social, and spiritual domains. It encourages individuals to identify a personal representative and to record and regularly review any preferences, so that their preferences can be taken into account should they at some point be unable to make their own decisions. (Rietjens et al. 2017 p.14)

This incorporates the three key elements described at the beginning of the chapter. They also set out the key components that should be covered in an ACP process:

- an individual's personal values and goals for future care
- clarification of goals and preferences for future medical treatment and care (including an exploration of whether these are realistic)
- discussing the option of completing an advance care directive and of appointing a personal representative, along with determining their role, as per local legal jurisdiction.

They recommended that individuals could "engage in ACP at any stage of their life, but that the ACP content can be more targeted when the individual's health condition worsens or as ageing progresses. In these circumstances, ACP conversations and documents should be updated regularly, as values and preferences may change over time" (Rietjens et al. 2017 p.14). This was the first world-wide attempt to get a consensus on what ACP and therefore be able to evaluate the process and understand what is needed to make it as effective as possible. Much of the literature on ACP so far is from North America, the UK, parts of Europe and Australasia. This partly reflects the development of palliative care services, but there may also be a cultural element around societal approaches to dying and death, as well as variations in how particular cultures are accepting of, or feel the need to plan out future decisions.

10.5 Ethical Issues in Advance Care Planning

Advance Care Planning is underpinned by an individual's values, beliefs and aspirations, set in the context of their family, community and the society they live in. As such, the ACP process potentially creates a number of ethical issues. Internationally, the most recognised ethics framework is the four principles of medical ethics (Beauchamp and Childress 2001):

- respect for the *Autonomy* of the patient
- acting for their *Beneficence*
- and avoiding harm: *Non-maleficence*
- while being fair to others in how we use resources: *Justice*

All four principles need to be in harmony with each other if a wise decision is to be made. One principle does not trump another. In recent times, autonomy has appeared to be a key driving principle in clinical decision making, as society reacts against perceived medical over-paternalism. However, autonomy refers not just to the patient, but also the health professional and requires the different expertise of both. Autonomy between individuals must still be balanced by the wider impact on society (justice). There are other approaches to the ethics of people's actions, for example focussing on people's duties (deontology), outcomes (consequentialist) or on the character of the individual making the decision (virtue ethics). Major ethical disagreements often arise because people are arguing from different points of view, for example focussing on the outcome when the other viewpoint is focussing on the action. Some health organisations have clinical ethics specialists or committees who can help to advise clinicians when faced with particular dilemmas.

10.5.1 Treatments and Interventions

A key aspect of ACP is deciding on the appropriateness of particular treatments and interventions. In a partnership between patients and their health professionals, patients are reliant on the expert advice they receive, tailored to their situation. That puts an onus on health professionals to consider carefully the intended benefit of an intervention versus the burdens or harm that the intervention may cause.

In palliative care, the potential benefits of a treatment are:

- Curing a disease
- Slowing down the disease process
- Preventing death
- Reducing disability or morbidity
- Providing symptom relief

Potential harms are treatments that:

- Cause side effects
- Cause illness, sometimes even death
- Waste excessive time or energy
- Provide "false hope"
- Prolong the dying phase when someone is suffering

In weighing these aspects up, the probability of the benefit and harm taking place also needs to be factored in, leading to a concept of the net benefit when all aspects have been weighed up. That net benefit is constantly changing, especially as people approach the end of their life. If there is no real prospect of achieving a benefit, pursuing the treatment is futile. Embarking on futile treatments exposes patients and their families to all the potential harms of a treatment for no reason. Different countries and cultures have a different perspective on their attitudes towards treatments that may be life prolonging, or futile. In some cultures, all treatments that may keep someone alive should be given. In other cultures, it is much more nuanced, with a balance between preserving life and not prolonging dying. More recently, some cultures have started to accept the argument that both preserving life and shortening life (physician physician-assisted suicide or euthanasia) where there is unresolved suffering can co-exist. In some states of the USA and western European counties both physician assisted suicide and euthanasia are now legal. That potentially allows individuals in those countries to include either as an intervention in the ACP process. In most countries, interventions aimed at shortening life are illegal and not allowed as part of the ACP or any other process.

Occasionally, in an ACP process, there will be disagreement between the patient and their family or health professional. Negotiation should resolve most issues, but if there is ongoing disagreement where a health professional feels a patient is either requesting an inappropriate treatment or refusing what seems an appropriate treatment, a second opinion should be sort. In most countries, the law supports patients to refuse any treatments they wish to, even life-prolonging ones, as long as they have full mental capacity to do so. Conversely, in most countries, patients are not legally entitled to any treatment they request if they are not clinically appropriate. Society has deemed that justice demands resources are used fairly and professionals determine that based on clinical benefit, risk and resources available. This idea links to the idea of "ordinary" and "extraordinary" treatments, proposed by Thomas Aquinas in the sixteenth century. Faced with significant advances in what medicine could do at the time, he proposed two tests to decide on the moral limits of trying to preserve life or health: the treatment needs to offer a reasonable hope of success and does not involve a physical or moral impossibility for the person involved. If both criteria are met, there is an obligation to treat as it is an "ordinary" treatment. If one or more condition is not met, the treatment would be considered "extraordinary" with no moral obligation to treat, and so can be done by choice.

10.5.2 Life Prolonging Treatments

There are particular potentially life prolonging treatments that may need particular consideration in the context of ACP: clinically assisted nutrition and hydration, ventilation and antibiotics. It is predictable that particular individuals may lose the ability to swallow or breathe independently, for example patients with neuromuscular disorders or towards the end of life in all patients with progressive illness.

Food and fluid create a particular challenge because they are part of normal life and fulfil basic needs of the body. Without them, life ceases which makes them particularly important for patients and families. Nevertheless, in people with advancing illness, the correct decision is not always clear. Clinically assisted nutrition in particular, is not without side effects and burdens. The evidence is mixed as to whether either treatment prolongs life (DoH 2007) so the anticipated benefit may need to be for something other than prolonging life, or in Aquinas' terms it would count as an "extraordinary" treatment. While clinically assisted hydration is less burdensome, it too can cause significant problems. Patients need to understand that loss of interest in food and drink is a part of the natural dying process and need not be medicalised, unless society determines that dying should be a medical process.

Ventilation may benefit some patients in respiratory failure in terms of managing breathlessness or prolonging their life. For many though, ventilation may serve to keep people alive for longer as their breathing continues to deteriorate, or do nothing but be burdensome. There are other common situations that pose similar issues for example supporting other organs or the use of antibiotics. At the heart of some of these decisions is the question about whether quality or quantity of life is more important for people, and whether potential treatments have a life prolonging effect or not. Understanding that helps professionals to interpret what is possible in a tailored way for patients. In drawing up a plan, if it is genuinely unclear whether to embark on a particular treatment, it makes clinical sense to either decide to assess the situation at the time when the clinical picture may be clearer, or to embark on a short treatment trial with the treatment withdrawn if it not achieving the desired net benefit especially if the burdens are significant, for example requiring a dying patient to be in hospital for a particular treatment.

DNACPR decisions have been considered from the perspective of making anticipatory clinical decisions. Like hydration, nutrition, ventilation and so on, cardiopulmonary resuscitation (CPR) in the event of a cardiac arrest is also an emotive issue. If not well handled, making a DNACPR decision can feel to patients as though professionals are just giving up on them, and allowing them to die when treatment could save them. The reality is that as a treatment, cardiopulmonary resuscitation is largely unsuccessful, especially in a palliative care group of patients (Sehatzadeh 2014). People often feel that deciding not to carry out resuscitation means that all forms of treatment will be, or will more likely be withdrawn. However, a DNACPR order specifically relates to the one treatment (CPR) and not to any other forms of treatment. A challenge in ACP is the ongoing change in a patient's situation. Even without an overt decision, it is expected that clinicians make appropriate decisions at the time. For example, CPR would not be a realistic treatment option in the context of a patient in the final stages of a terminal illness where death is imminent and unavoidable because it is futile and inappropriate. If CPR is unlikely to re-start the patient's circulation or breathing, CPR should not be attempted.

In an ideal world, DNACPR discussions and decisions are an important part of the ACP process. For most other clinical decisions, there is no requirement for health professionals to discuss treatments that are considered futile. However, the UK court set out a legal position on the involvement of patients and their families in the decision making around DNACPR decisions (Royal Courts of Justice 2014).

Healthcare professionals must consult with patients (or relatives and carers if the patient lacks mental capacity) about any decision to put a DNACPR order in place. Article 8 of the European Court of Human Rights guarantees a patient's right to respect for private and family life. Failure to consult about DNACPR decisions may breach this right and a doctor's common law duties (MacCormick et al. 2018). The only exceptions to this ruling are situations where it is not appropriate to discuss, perhaps if that discussion would cause physical or psychological harm to the patient or where it is not practical to discuss the decision, for example where there is a sudden change in condition. Clinical futility is not considered an acceptable reason for not discussing a DNACPR decision. These issues are very topical and case law is evolving. It remains to be seen whether other countries would apply the same interpretation.

There is a danger that court cases can lead to health professionals practising in a defensive way, to avoid making difficult decisions, or evade conversations about difficult issues. DNACPR discussions are part of a spectrum of decisions that may need to be addressed in a context of a patient deteriorating progressively and in the dying phase of their disease.

10.5.3 Capacity

Mental capacity is an area that is integral to the process of ACP. Capacity is not an all or nothing phenomenon. People may have capacity for some decisions but not for others. Loss of capacity may be temporary or permanent and if it is temporary, every effort should be made to support an individual to regain their capacity. Dehydration, confusion and depression are common temporary causes of loss of capacity. Individual countries define how capacity should be assessed, often backed up by relevant legislation. In principle, capacity is about being able to understand the decision that needs to be made; being able to understand and weigh up the benefits, burdens and consequences of particular decisions; and being able to retain and communicate that decision.

Capacity is important to ACP in a number of ways:

- While discussions about the present and future can meaningfully take place with people who lack full capacity, those discussions may lose full meaning depending on the aspect of capacity lost.
- Patients must have full capacity to make valid decisions as part of the ACP process. If those decisions were made at a time when they did not have capacity, the decisions lose validity.
- Any formal decisions that have been made ahead of time only come in to force if a patient loses mental capacity for the particular decision. Even if a formal document is in place, it does not apply if a patient retains capacity.

10.6 Does ACP Work?

ACP has the potential to empower patients to regain some control of their lives through understanding more about their situation, discussing potential options and making specific plans. When ACP takes place, the interactions between patients and health professionals improve, patient satisfaction increases and more formal specific plans are likely to be made (Brinkman-Stoppelenburg et al. 2014, Houben et al. 2014).

A big challenge in assessing the effectiveness of the ACP process is the variation in how it is carried out, and with what purpose. That makes it hard to make comparisons with different datasets. While initially ACP may have focussed on supporting people who may lose capacity within a legislative framework, it is now a wider process to encourage all patients to think about their health and plan the future. For policy planners, it is tempting to use ACP as a tool to reduce the pressure on hospital beds (and to judge success based on that) because people who make informed decisions about the future tend to choose less expensive/intensive care (Mulley et al. 2012). That approach is flawed because ACP is a process, not a moment in time decision. It will be hard to truly measure the effectiveness of ACP until the purpose is agreed. Apart from the purpose of ACP, another challenge is whether there are sophisticated enough measures to effectively capture a complex process of ongoing conversation, reflection and refinement. Otherwise, the temptation is to use crude outcome measures which do not capture the essence of ACP, such as document completion or whether a conversation has taken place, however good or limited.

10.7 Final Thoughts

ACP has, at heart, evolved in to a social movement, one that seeks to get people to talk about all aspects of their situation, including their changing health, their hopes and fears, and, through working with health professionals, to make plans to address some anticipated problems. For most people, opportunities to find out more about their health and their choices or options are both empowering and positive. Currently, there is a clear gap in what patients would like to know and what information they are receiving. Being informed about and discussing their health seems to be a bigger priority for patients than making definite decisions. For many patients, being able to talk about this is therapeutic and they see no reason to take the process beyond that. Perhaps our communication with patients needs to mature to give them the tools they need, before we can truly realise the full benefits of ACP and deliver more formal plans that are meaningful in delivering what patients aspire to.

When delivering clear plans, ACP may deliver significant cost savings as people opt for less medicalisation of the dying process, but may put people off the process if that is perceived to be the driving factor: real choice or one that is financially driven. Focussing on the plan or the output is much easier than trying to improve the conversations, and is more easily measurable. Regular ongoing dialogue about the situation, prognosis, concerns and options is important as people's views change. What is important to an individual evolves- autonomy may not be that important to people at the end of their life.

For health professionals, some knowledge is needed about the framework and legislation in their own country around ACP. In particular the approach to offering or withholding/withdrawing treatments needs to be culturally sensitive and fit with national guidelines and laws. The most important aspect is the communication skills required to address the present situation, converse about the future in a way that is supportive and realistic without extinguishing hope; and to talk through potential treatment options in a way that is tailored to the individual and their family.

If that is able to happen, ACP can be one of the most powerful tools we have to empower vulnerable patients. Without these skills, it is a blunt tool that risks significant harm through insensitive communication.

References

Beauchamp, T., and J. Childress. 2001. *Principles of biomedical ethics*. 5th ed. New York: Oxford University Press.

Brinkman-Stoppelenburg, A., J. Rietjens, and A. van der Heide. 2014. The effects of advance care planning on end-of-life care: A systematic review. *Palliative Medicine* 28 (8): 1000–1025.

Churm, D. 2016. *Advance care planning in Parkinson's disease*. M.D. Thesis, Newcastle University.

Davies, A., J. Todd, F. Bailey, et al. 2016. Good concordance between patients and their non-professional carers about factors associated with a 'good death' and other important end-of-life decisions. *BMJ Supportive & Palliative Care*. Published Online First: 17 May 2016. https://doi.org/10.1136/bmjspcare-2015-001085.

Department of Health. 2007. *Improving nutritional care. A Joint action plan from the Department of Health and Nutrition Summit stakeholders*. DOH: Leeds.

Detering, K., A. Hancock, M. Reade, and W. Silvester. 2010. The impact of advance care planning on end of life care in elderly patients: Randomised controlled trial. *BMJ* 340: c1345.

Drought, T., and B. Koenig. 2002. "Choice" in end-of-life decision making: Researching fact or fiction? *The Gerontologist*. 42 (3): 114–128. https://doi.org/10.1093/geront/42.suppl_3.114.

e-ELCA. 2010. *E-learning for healthcare: e-End of life care for all*. London: Department of Health. http://www.e-lfh.org.uk/projects/e-elca/index.html.

Fritz, Z., A.-M. Slowther, and G. Perkins. 2017. Resuscitation policy should focus on the patient, not the decision. *BMJ*. 356: j813.

Goodridge, D. 2006. COPD as a life-limiting illness: Advance care planning. *Topics in Advanced Practice Nursing* 6: 1–8.

Heffner, J., P. Nieterr, and C. Barbieri. 2000. Pleural fluid pH as a predictor of survival for patients with malignant pleural effusions. *Chest* 117 (1): 79–86. https://doi.org/10.1378/chest.117.1.79.

Houben, C., M. Spruit, M. Groenen, E. Wouters, and D. Janssen. 2014. Efficacy of advance care planning: A systematic review and meta-analysis. *Journal of the American Medical Directors Association* 15 (7): 477–489.

Lamont, E., and M. Siegler. 2000. Paradoxes in cancer patients' advance care planning. *Journal of Palliative Medicine*. 3 (1): 27–35.

MacCormick, F., C. Emmett, P. Paes, and J. Hughes. 2018. Resuscitation decisions at the end of life: Medical views and the juridification of practice. *Journal of Medical Ethics*. 44: 376–383.

MacPherson, A., C. Walshe, V. O'Donnell, and A. Vyas. 2013. The views of patients with severe chronic obstructive pulmonary disease on advance care planning: A qualitative study. *Palliative Medicine.* 27 (3): 265–272. https://doi.org/10.1177/0269216312440606.

Mulley, A., C. Trimble, and G. Elwyn. 2012. *Patients' preferences matter: Stop the silent misdiagnosis.* London: King's Fund.

NHS North East. 2011. *Deciding right: An integrated approach to making care decisions in advance with children, young people and adults.* NHS North East.

Paes, P., and C. O'Neill. 2012. Treatment escalation plans – A tool to aid end of life decision making? *BMJ Supportive & Palliative Care.* 2: A60.

Pautex, S., F. Herrmann, and G. Zulian. 2008. Role of advance directives in palliative care units: A prospective study. *Palliative Medicine.* 22 (7): 835–841. https://doi.org/10.1177/0269216308094336.

Reynolds, K., L. Hanson, M. Henderson, et al. 2008. End-of-life care in nursing home settings: Do race or age matter? *Palliative and Supportive Care.* 6 (1): 21–27.

Rietjens, J., R. Sudore, M. Connolly, et al. 2017. Definition and recommendations for advance care planning: An international consensus supported by the European Association for Palliative Care. *Lancet Oncology.* 18: e543–e551.

Robinson, L., C. Dickinson, N. Rousseau, et al. 2011. A systematic review of the effectiveness of advance care planning interventions for people with cognitive impairment and dementia. *Age and Ageing.* 41 (2): 263–269.

Royal Courts of Justice. 2014. *Tracey versus Cambridge University Hospitals NHS Foundation Trust and others.* London: Royal Courts of Justice. https://www.judiciary.gov.uk/wp-content/uploads/2014/2006/tracey-approved.pdf.

Sehatzadeh, S. 2014. Cardiopulmonary resuscitation in patients with terminal illness: An evidence-based analysis. *Ontario Health Technology Assessment Series.* 14 (15): 1–38.

Smucker, W., P. Ditto, et al. 1993. Elderly outpatients respond favorably to a physician-initiated advance directive discussion. *Journal of the American Board of Family Practitioners.* 6 (5): 473–482.

Teno, J., A. Gruneir, Z. Schwartz, et al. 2007. Association between advance directives and quality of end-of-life care: A national study. *Journal of the American Geriatrics Society.* 55: 189–194.

Virdun, C., T. Luckett, P. Davidson, et al. 2015. Dying in the hospital setting: A systematic review of quantitative studies identifying the elements of end-of-life care that patients and their families rank as being most important. *Palliative Medicine.* 29 (9): 774–796.

Wagner, D., D. Riopelle, K. Steckart, et al. 2010. Provider communication and patient understanding of life-limiting illness and their relationship to patient communication of treatment preferences. *Journal of Pain and Symptom Management.* 39 (3): 527–534.

Chapter 11
Importance of Training

Francesca Pistoia

Abstract This chapter addresses the importance of a proper training for health care professionals facing end of life care issues. A significant psychological and moral distress is associated with the management both of dying patients and of patients with progressive degenerative diseases without hope of definitive healing. The above distress involves not only physicians working in the Intensive Care Units (ICU) but also various health care figures acting in residential long-term care settings, with difficulties being peculiar to each specific context. The chapter address the main concern faced by Health Care Assistants in End-of-Life Care and highlights the importance of a preparatory training allowing the professionals to acquire specific skills and coping strategies, which are essential for an effective and evidenced-based management of the patients. The need for a specific training is even more evident if we consider the progressive aging of the population, with a growing need for End-of-Life Care assessments and a worldwide social and psychological burden. Nevertheless, the necessity of a specific training addressing end of life issues is still underestimated with medical students being mainly involved in saving lives and little or nothing trained in facing patients' death.

Keywords Training · Specialist palliative care · Generalist palliative care · Moral judgment

11.1 Introduction

This chapter addresses the importance of a proper training for health care professionals facing end of life care issues. A significant psychological and moral distress is associated with the management both of dying patients and of patients with

F. Pistoia (✉)
Neurological Institute, Department of Applied Clinical Sciences and Biotechnology, University of L'Aquila, L'Aquila, Italy
e-mail: eliana.close@qut.edu.au

P. Mallia et al. (eds.), *Challenges to the Global Issue of End of Life Care*, Advancing Global Bioethics 17, https://doi.org/10.1007/978-3-030-86386-9_11

progressive degenerative diseases without hope of definitive healing. The above distress involves not only physicians working in the Intensive Care Units (ICU) but also various health care figures acting in residential long-term care settings, with difficulties being peculiar to each specific context. The chapter address the main concern faced by Health Care Assistants in End-of-Life Care and highlights the importance of a preparatory training allowing the professionals to acquire specific skills and coping strategies, which are essential for an effective and evidenced-based management of the patients. The need for a specific training is even more evident if we consider the progressive aging of the population, with a growing need for End-of-Life Care assessments and a worldwide social and psychological burden. Nevertheless, the necessity of a specific training addressing end of life issues is still underestimated with medical students being mainly involved in saving lives and little or nothing trained in facing patients' death.

> *I learned about a lot of things in medical school, but mortality wasn't one of them... our textbooks had almost nothing on aging or frailty or death. How the process unfolds, how people experience the end of their lives, and how it affects those around them seemed beside the point. The way we saw it... the purpose of medical schooling was to teach us how to save lives, not how to tend to their demise.* – Being Mortal: Medicine and What Matters in the End, Atul Gawande.

11.2 Training in Bein- Involved

Even physicians trained to face end of life conditions, when encountering with extremely suffering patients and their caregivers, may be stunned. This condition has been brilliantly reported by Camus in his novel *The Plague*, where the author describes a physician managing patients with unbearable suffering and hopeless prognosis. Even if the author refers to a specific condition, that is a pest epidemic, the description of the uncertainty and the fear experienced by the physician called to face the disaster well sums it up the psychological and moral distress that health professionals face in end-of-life settings. Several studies investigated the moral distress experienced by physicians engaged with patients suffering from serious illnesses. Moral distress was originally described by Jameton (1984) as *the feeling arising when one knows the right thing to do, but perceived or prevailing institutional constraints prevent the right action*. Further reflections led to incorporating the concept of moral dilemma, that occurs when *someone does not know what is ethically right, but has to make a decision* into the construct of moral distress (O'Donnell et al. 2008). Usually moral distress arises in those situations in which the health professional cannot share choices with the patient in front of him. This occurs, for instance, in the case of behaviourally unresponsive patients, suffering from coma, vegetative state or minimally conscious state. Such patients don't show any purposeful action and functional communication, and, as a consequence, no dialogue is possible between them and the physician engaged in their care (Sarà and Pistoia 2010; Zylberman et al. 2016). Therefore, the health professional is often required to decide autonomously, or with the help of relatives and caregivers, about ethically difficult situations regarding the level of care, the need of futile or disproportional treatment, the demand for palliative care and the necessity to carry out painful procedures in patients with extremely poor recovery chances. Similarly, moral distress can be experienced when facing patients in whom treatment strategies are at high risk of being ineffective due to the severity of the underlying disease. In this venue, a recent study investigated the professional quality of life in physicians and nurses at a tertiary care hospital and suggested that the events which mainly contribute to the moral distress of professionals lie with working with critical care patients and providing care that seems ineffective (Austin et al. 2017). Similarly, decisions to maintain or to limit life-prolonging treatments are associated with a high degree of moral distress, especially when managing advanced cancer inpatients or patients with chronic long-term diseases (Mehlis et al. 2018). Moral distress is also at the highest level when managing children with severe diseases (Sandeberg et al. 2020; Sandeberg et al. 2017) especially when parents have unrealistic expectation of health care. Empathy, compassion and care have been described as the main characteristics that health professional should have or develop to properly address these conditions. Empathy is defined as the adequate understanding of the inner processes of the patient concerning his health-related problems (Gelhaus 2012a, b) while compassion refers to the attitude to share sadness feeling with suffering patients (Gelhaus 2012a, b). Empathy and compassion are the prerequisite to plan proper patient-tailored care (Gelhaus 2013). Ethical guideline and specific training are necessary in order to learn proper coping strategies in handling complex and stressful end-of-life conditions. Implementing emotional wellness activities (e.g., empowerment, opportunity for open dialog regarding ethical issues, policy making involvement) may be of help in training (Austin et al. 2017).

11.3 Training in Developing Competency in Moral Judgement

The development of moral judgment competency is essential to face complex situations where a moral dilemma arises because the clinician is not sure of what is ethically right to do but he has to make a decision about it. Education at university should prepare students, destined to work in the health field, in the inner process of moral judgment development. However, unexpected findings on this topic came from studies investigating the effects of medical education on moral development by comparing first and fourth/fifth year medical students with respect to moral reasoning (Lind 2000). The majority of these studies concluded that medical education does not contribute to students' moral development, as upward changes in moral development are not observed in function of the progressive academic growing of the involved subjects. The observed tendency is that medical students, during their academic course, get a highly sophisticated technical training but not the moral tools, which are necessary to deal with complex situations and moral dilemmas. Surprisingly, some studies showed that students ever regress with respect to their moral judgement repertoire as academic career goes on, and that they are ultimately much more concentrated on the technical aspects of their profession than on moral issues. This profile could have a growing trend if we think about how much health care professionals are today absorbed by medical technology across all scientific disciplines, with the risk of shelving the human side of medicine, based on dialogue and relationship with the patients. An example of how technology can be misleading and generate ethical dilemmas is the following: recently, patients with behaviourally unresponsive state (named as vegetative state or unresponsive wakefulness syndrome) have been investigated by functional Magnetic Resonance Imaging (fMRI). While undergoing fMRI, patients were asked to imagine playing tennis or moving around the rooms of their home: in some patients, the researchers identified the same brain activation patterns which can be recognized in healthy subjects, thus suggesting that technology provides a new mean for detecting conscious awareness when a standard clinical approach is unable to provide that information (Owen et al. 2007; Sarà et al. 2008; Sarà and Pistoia 2012). This evidence is undoubtedly of great help for the science because it paves the way for new approaches to investigate the issue of unconsciousness in behaviourally unresponsive patients. However, at the same time, it raises important ethical questions, not least the need to explain to relatives why patients, whose cerebral patterns seem to be intact, do not interact in any way with them and the environment (Sarà and Pistoia 2010). In this case, it is the technology itself to raise an ethical dilemma that clinicians are not able to handle and resolve. Hence the confusion that inevitably arises at the patient's bedside, that it is difficult to be managed if clinicians are not trained to use and implement moral reasoning. This and other conditions prompt reflection on the importance to train the ability for moral reasoning, starting from the years of university study.

11.4 Training in Communication

Communicating in an effective and empathic way is the prerequisite to carry out good palliative care strategies. The complexity of diseases requiring palliative care makes communication with patients and caregivers more difficult and challenging. The aim of communication is describing the severity of the disease and sharing information on prognosis, management and, eventually, end-of-life decisions. The first step in the communication process is to make the patient and his relatives informed of the complexity of the situation in which they find themselves: it is a difficult circumstance because the patient often does not have the cultural tools to understand the mechanisms underlying the disease and the natural history of the pathology which he is suffering from. It follows that he can react by completely relying on the physician who is managing him or reacting with detachment and distrust to the situation. The later step is sharing information on prognosis *quoad vitam*, *quoad valetudinem* and *quoad functionem* that is explaining to the patient the likelihood of survival, recovery and impairment of functions. Appropriateness and effectiveness of communication skills depend on the clinical scenarios we are involved in. For instance, talking about survival may be particularly challenging for patients with cancer, especially those in a young age. Even more difficult may be establishing and communicating a prognosis on survival in patients with severe acquired brain injuries leading to disorders of consciousness: in this case, the physician cannot establish with absolute certainty what the natural history of the disease will be and he is not able to answer the legitimate questions of relatives about the chances for recovery. In fact, even in cases where the chances are exceedingly small, the prognosis should be established in a probabilistic way, as physicians may experience unexpected recoveries even long after the initial acquired brain injury. In these cases, sharing information on prognosis with relatives and caregivers may be very difficult, as physicians move in a grey zone where doubts and controversies influence care, management and end-of-care making decisions. Similar difficulties may occur when there is the need of communicating prognosis for patients with other neurological conditions as dementia, Parkinson disease and amyotrophic lateral sclerosis: in such cases, the physician is reasonably aware of what the clinical course of the disease will be but he may experience a sense of helplessness because he is handling patients with progressive degenerative diseases without hope of healing. Different conditions are those where the disorder does not imply a short-term risk for survival but it compromises the general functions of the patient: an example is represented by progressive heart or respiratory failure where the quality of life of patients is highly impaired and the patients have to be educated to face daily difficulties. A separate case is represented by the communication needs of neonatologists within the Neonatal Intensive Care Units (NICU), who are exposed to complex situations where a clear and empathic communication with the family is the prerequisite to properly manage critically ill infants. Nevertheless, available evidence on training in this context shows that the majority of neonatologists does not receive formal training targeted at communication skills (Henner and Boss 2017; Boss et al. 2009). The lack of training often results in confusion and moral distress not only for patients and relatives but also for physicians who feel themselves inadequate to match others' needs. Therefore, communication is a core competence to handle vulnerable patients and vulnerable families: so a structured end-of-life care curriculum should include a specific training in holding difficult conservations in each specific end of life care setting. In fact, available evidence suggests that a proper communication increases the concordance degree between patients/caregivers and health care professionals and improves patient's satisfaction with care (Brighton and Bristowe 2016; You et al. 2014). Despite this, the percentage of patients with critical illness, which report not having ever discussed end-of-life care issues with clinicians, is very high (Brighton and Bristowe 2016). The major barrier to communication is just the feeling of inadequacy experienced by not trained clinicians in discussing end of life care issues together with the lack of timely communication windows in dealing with such problems along the trajectory of each disease. We can encounter a series of pitfalls when establishing a proper communication with patients (Back 2020). The deficiencies being recognized can be easily found in patients with cancer as well as in other clinical scenarios, all characterized by the lack of a definitive healing. The continuous efforts of clinicians in fostering the clinician-patient relationship may be partially invalidated by the tendency to introduce palliative care as an end-of-life service rather than as a supportive care, the inclination to undercut hope or to abandon the patient near the end, and the practice of not including other team members when communicating with patients and caregivers. Similarly, where there is a need of discussing serious news, the main pitfalls include the tendency to proceed without before assessing what the patient already knows and to use a medical jargon, which is unfamiliar to the patient. Moreover, in this context, the ability to capture the emotional reactions of patients, as expressed by language and nonverbal behaviours, is the prerequisite to further dealing with their emotions. Other difficulties in communication may arise from the necessity to prepare patients for the future, informing them about mortality and survival: the clinician often tends to be vague even if the patient explicitly asks about dying, which results in a misleading communication (Back 2020). Finally, clinicians often fail in involving family caregivers during conservations, thus underestimating their concerns and involvement in the clinical course of the disease. All these factors represent barriers to a correct communication and should be overcome by timely training healthcare professionals in handling challenging clinical situations starting from communication itself.

11.5 Training in Early Identification of Palliative Care Needs

Palliative care is defined by the World Health Organisation as the approach that improves the quality of life of patients and their families facing the problem associated with life- threatening illness, through the prevention and relief of suffering by means of early identification and impeccable assessment and treatment of pain and other problems, physical, psychosocial and spiritual (World Health Organization 2013). Aims of palliative care include providing relief from pain, affirming life and regards dying as a normal process, intending neither to hasten or postpone death and integrating the psychological and spiritual aspects of patient care. One of the first skills that professionals involved in palliative care should acquire is the ability to early identify patients who would benefit from palliative approaches. The core question we have to reply is: "Do all the patients with advanced or incurable illness or nearing the end of life need palliative support?" Unfortunately, it is unlikely that all the patients who are approaching to death receive a comprehensive assessment aimed at evaluating their needs in terms of palliative care. So clinicians should learn how to identify patients with the most relevant palliative needs. Available scientific evidence suggests that this identification almost never happens in a timely manner and patients receive palliative care very late in the clinical course of their diseases, when they are just close to death. This occurs because palliative care often starts when healthcare professionals realize themselves that patients might die in the foreseeable future, but in multiple circumstances there is a mismatch between the moment of physcians foreseeing death and the moment of patients' actual death. This mismatch is maximum when clinicians are managing non-competent patients, that are behaviourally unresponsive patients or patients with intellectual disabilities, due to a restriction in their communication repertoire (Vrijmoeth et al. 2016). Consequences of the late recognition of palliative care needs include the following: a high percentage of patients who wish to die at home end up dying in the hospital; not all the patients receive the best symptom management or are prescribed with inappropriate treatments; family and caregivers are not properly supported from a psychological point of view (Teike Lüthi et al. 2020). On this venue, there is a general consensus on the fact that palliative care should be initiated as early as possible along the clinical course of the disease. Therefore there is the need of specific tools and skills enabling clinicians to early recognize end-of-life conditions as the prerequisite to properly manage them. The so-called surprise question, worded as "Would you be surprised if your patient died in the next one month?" has been recently proposed as a reliable and easy tool to capture patients that are more than a year from death and are potentially candidate for receiving palliative care (Downar et al. 2019; Ouchi et al. 2019). The use of this question prompts clinicians to reflect on the real trajectory of the disease of their patients, in order to timely start palliative care. This is particularly relevant when facing behaviourally unresponsive patients, whose palliative needs are at risk of being underestimated and being unmet, due to their inability to communicate. Just these patients have multiple sources of possible pain and discomfort, including the presence of muscular spasticity, pressure ulcers, traumatic fractures and heterotopic ossification and the presence of life-supporting devices (tracheostomy, feeding tube, central venous catheter, percutaneous endoscopic gastrostomy, urinary catheter etc.). Investigating pain in this category of patients is very challenging and we usually infer the presence of any clinical discomfort from indirect signs showed by the patients (Pistoia et al. 2015a, b, 2016). This the prerequisite for the use of the Nociception Coma Scale which investigates the presence of non verbal signs of pain as the first step for providing relief (Schnakers et al. 2010) In this respect, the use of other scales assessing the presence of medical comorbidities and of complications may be of further help in identifying those patients who are more likely to suffer from physical pain (Pistoia et al. 2015a, b, 2019; Scarponi et al. 2019).

11.6 Training for Inter-Professional Work and Civic Engagement

A specific training for health professionals aimed at developing palliative care core competencies is worldwide desired. The most pressing need lies with the idea of integrating palliative care with the other medical disciplines overlapping it, such as oncology, neurology and geriatric medicine. In fact, the prerequisite to obtain an effective educational program for health care professionals starts from encouraging the implementation of an *Inter-Professional Model of Patient Care*. This model, which has the advantage to be centred on the patient and his global well-being rather than on the disease itself, implies the stable collaboration among different health care professionals from different disciplines, such as intensive care physicians, oncologists, neurologists, pneumologists, nurses, speech therapists, social workers, spiritual care providers, psychologists, counselors and figures belonging to other fields. The stable collaboration between these professionals triggers a virtuous circle in which the result is not the sum of the activities of the individual operators but their product, leading to the greatest care satisfaction for the patient and caregivers. Obviously, the objectives of palliative therapy are different according to the underlying pathology, so that an health care professional involved in palliative care should learn to collaborate with the other figures and, at the same time, to develop specific competencies which depend on the individual characteristics of patients he is managing.

In this venue, an integrated public health approach to palliative care has been recently proposed: this approach implies the stable and bidirectional collaboration between specialist and generalist palliative care workers, with the coupled involvement of compassionate communities, working in association with key civic institutions (Abel et al. 2018). This organization follows the principle of social justice, according to which everyone has the right to benefit from palliative care regardless of age, background, diagnosis and prognosis. The first step in planning this approach lies with establishing the specific competencies of specialist and generalist palliative care workers: although the boundary between these two areas may be blurred, establishing which skills are needed in each of the two categories is essential to develop effective training program for future health care professionals. Usually, specialist palliative care has the objective to manage more complex conditions like neuropathic pain and several medical complications including those favoured by prolonged hospitalisation and bed immobilization whereas generalist palliative care address the problems which raise in daily clinical care and in the social sphere of end-of life patients. There is a wide variability across countries in the training programs of workers involved in specialist and generalist palliative care: in some countries, specialist palliative care represents a separate medical specialty while, in others, it simply summarizes a series of skills, which are progressively acquired by other specialists in the course of their training and professional course. On the other hand, in most of countries, generalist palliative care is not a separate discipline but it involves all health and social care professionals who deliver care to patients who are dying, while providing social and psychological support to their families (Abel et al. 2018). General practitioners, nursing staff, social workers and psychologists are the figures mainly involved in the field of generalist palliative care across all countries. Both generalist and palliative care professionals have the duty and the interest to interact with the community and the institutions, in order to provide their technical contribution to improve the integrated public health approach and to reduce the recognized barriers of access to palliative care. The close partnership among all the members and structures of the palliative care network is the only way to properly address the needs of patients and their families. An example of the above collaborative partnership is offered by an innovative model of a home-like environment for people in chronic vegetative and minimally conscious state, named *Casa*

Iride, which has recently been implemented in Italy: it is a non-medicalized cohousing community where patients, although not being considered terminally ill, receive all the support they need (Zylberman et al. 2016). At the same time, the caregivers of patients share a place with other people with similar challenges, thus becoming more aware of a condition, which is difficult to understand, and learning to cope with it. This triggers a virtuous cycle also from a social and economic point of view with direct and indirect costs being reduced, as the care flow of patients through intensive care units and intensive rehabilitation wards is not delayed by a lack of post discharge services and family members can maintain their productivity at work (Zylberman et al. 2016).

References

Abel, J., A. Kellehear, and A. Karapliagou. 2018 Apr. Palliative care-the new essentials. *Annals of Palliative Medicine* 7 (Suppl 2): S3–S14.

Austin, C.L., R. Saylor, and P.J. Finley. 2017 Jul. Moral distress in physicians and nurses: Impact on professional quality of life and turnover. *Psychological Trauma* 9 (4): 399–406.

Back, A.L. 2020 Mar 20. Patient-clinician communication issues in palliative care for patients with advanced cancer. *Journal of Clinical Oncology* 38 (9): 866–876.

Boss, R.D., N. Hutton, P.K. Donohue, and R.M. Arnold. 2009 Sep. Neonatologist training to guide family decision making for critically ill infants. *Archives of Pediatrics & Adolescent Medicine* 163 (9): 783–788.

Brighton, L.J., and K. Bristowe. 2016 Aug. Communication in palliative care: Talking about the end of life, before the end of life. *Postgraduate Medical Journal* 92 (1090): 466–470.

Downar, J., P. Wegier, and P. Tanuseputro. 2019 Sep. Early identification of people who would benefit from a palliative approach-moving from surprise to routine. *JAMA Netw Open* 2 (9): e1911146.

Gawande, A. 2014. *Being mortal: Medicine and what matters in the end*. Metropolitan Books/Henry Holt and Company.

Gelhaus, P. 2012a May. The desired moral attitude of the physician: (I) empathy. *Medicine, Health Care, and Philosophy* 15 (2): 103–113.

Gelhaus, P. 2012b Nov. The desired moral attitude of the physician: (II) compassion. *Medicine, Health Care, and Philosophy* 15 (4): 397–410.

Gelhaus, P. 2013 May. The desired moral attitude of the physician: (III) care. *Medicine, Health Care, and Philosophy* 16 (2): 125–139.

Jameton, A. 1984. *Nursing practice, the ethical issues*. Englewood Cliffs: Prentice Hall.

O'Donnell, P., A. Farrar, K. BrintzenhofeSzoc, A.P. Conrad, M. Danis, C. Grady, C. Taylor, and C.M. Ulrich. 2008. Predictors of ethical stress, moral action and job satisfaction in health care social workers. *Social Work in Health Care* 46 (3): 29–51.

Henner, N., and R.D. Boss. 2017 Mar. Neonatologist training in communication and palliative care. *Seminars in Perinatology* 41 (2): 106–110.

You, J.J., P. Dodek, F. Lamontagne, J. Downar, T. Sinuff, X. Jiang, A.G. Day, and D.K. Heyland. 2014 Dec 9. For the ACCEPT Study Team and the Canadian Researchers at the End of Life Network (CARENET). What really matters in end-of-life discussions? Perspectives of patients in hospital with serious illness and their families. *CMAJ* 186 (18): E679–E687.

Lind, G. 2000. Moral regression in medical students and their learning environment. *Revista Brasileira De Educacao Medica* 24 (3): 24–33.

Mehlis, K., E. Bierwirth, K. Laryionava, F.H.A. Mumm, W. Hiddemann, and P. Heußner. 2018 Dec. Winkler EC High prevalence of moral distress reported by oncologists and oncology nurses in end-of-life decision making. *Psycho-Oncology* 27 (12): 2733–2739.

Ouchi, K., Strout, T., Haydar, S., et al. 2019. Association of emergency clinicians' assessment of mortality risk with actual 1-month mortality among older adults admitted to the hospital. *JAMA Netw Open* 2 (9): e1911139.

Owen, A.M., M.R. Coleman, M. Boly, M.H. Davis, S. Laureys, and J.D. Pickard. 2007 Aug. Using functional magnetic resonance imaging to detect covert awareness in the vegetative state. *Archives of Neurology* 64 (8): 1098–1102.

Pistoia, F., S. Sacco, J. Stewart, M. Sarà, and A. Carolei. 2016 Oct. Disorders of consciousness: Painless or painful conditions?-Evidence from neuroimaging studies. *Brain Sciences* 8: 6(4).

Pistoia, F., S. Sacco, M. Sarà, M. Franceschini, and A. Carolei. 2015a Jan. Intrathecal baclofen: Effects on spasticity, pain, and consciousness in disorders of consciousness and locked-in syndrome. *Current Pain and Headache Reports* 19 (1): 466.

Pistoia, F., S. Sacco, M. Franceschini, M. Sarà, C. Pistarini, B. Cazzulani, I. Simonelli, P. Pasqualetti, and A. Carolei. 2015b May 15. Comorbidities: A key issue in patients with disorders of consciousness. *Journal of Neurotrauma* 32 (10): 682–688.

Pistoia, F., A. Carolei, Y.G. Bodien, S. Greenfield, S. Kaplan, S. Sacco, C. Pistarini, A. Casalena, A. De Tanti, B. Cazzulani, G. Bellaviti, M. Sarà, and J. Giacino. 2019 Oct 17. The comorbidities coma scale (CoCoS): Psychometric properties and clinical usefulness in patients with disorders of consciousness. *Frontiers in Neurology* 10: 1042.

Sandeberg, M., C. Bartholdson, and P. Pergert. 2020 Jan 13. Important situations that capture moral distress in paediatric oncology. *BMC Medical Ethics* 21 (1): 6.

Sandeberg, M., M. Wenemark, C. Bartholdson, K. Lützén, and P. Pergert. 2017 Feb 20. To change or not to change – translating and culturally adapting the paediatric version of the moral distress scale-revised (MDS-R). *BMC Medical Ethics* 18 (1): 14.

Sarà, M., F. Pistoia, G. Cernera, and S. Sacco. 2008 Mar. The consciousness dilemma: Feel or feel of feeling? *Arch Neurol* 65 (3): 418.

Sarà, M., and F. Pistoia. 2012 May 5. Bedside detection of awareness in the vegetative state. *Lancet* 379 (9827): 1702–1703.

Sarà M., and F. Pistoia. 2010 Apr. Defining consciousness: Lessons from patients and modern techniques. *Journal of Neurotrauma* 27 (4): 771–773.

Teike Lüthi, F., M. Bernard, M. Beauverd, C. Gamondi, A.S. Ramelet, and G.D. Borasio. 2020 Feb 12. IDentification of patients in need of general and specialised PALLiative care (ID-PALL©): Item generation, content and face validity of a new interprofessional screening instrument. *BMC Palliative Care* 19 (1): 19.

Scarponi, F., M. Zampolini, C. Zucchella, S. Bargellesi, C. Fassio, F. Pistoia, and M. Bartolo. 2019 Apr. C.I.R.C.LE study group. Identifying clinical complexity in patients affected by severe acquired brain injury in neurorehabilitation: A cross sectional survey. *European Journal of Physical and Rehabilitation Medicine* 55 (2): 191–198.

Schnakers, C., C. Chatelle, A. Vanhaudenhuyse, S. Majerus, D. Ledoux, M. Boly, M.A. Bruno, P. Boveroux, A. Demertzi, G. Moonen, and S. Laureys. 2010 Feb. The nociception coma scale: A new tool to assess nociception in disorders of consciousness. *Pain* 148 (2): 215–219.

Vrijmoeth, C., M.G. Christians, D.A. Festen, M. Groot, A. van der Heide, C.C. van der Rijt, M. Tonino, and M.A. Echteld. 2016 Nov. Physician-reported symptoms and interventions in people with intellectual disabilities approaching end of life. *Journal of Palliative Medicine* 19 (11): 1142–1147.

World Health Organization. (2013). WHO Definition of Palliative Care. Retrieved from http://www.who.int/cancer/palliative/definition/en

Zylberman, R., A. Carolei, S. Sacco, P. Mallia, and F. Pistoia. 2016 Jan. An innovative model of a home-like environment for people in vegetative and minimally conscious states. *Neurohospitalist* 6 (1): 14–19.

Chapter 12
Palliative Sedation – Is It a Real Dilemma?

Nathan Emmerich

Abstract Given the extensive literature on the topic it seems clear that palliative sedation raises particularly challenging ethical questions. Nevertheless, Savulescu and Radcliffe-Richards (Anaesthesia. https://doi.org/10.1111/anae.14635, 2019) have recently suggested that patients not only have a right to be given analgesia and sedation in response to pain but also have a right to be rendered unconscious if and when this is required to effectively manage their pain. This essay follows a similar line of reasoning and suggests that the extensive ethical analysis of palliative sedation may result in an overabundance of ethical caution that has the potential to lead to patients suffering needlessly. Thus I offer a corrective and argue that the clinical needs of dying patients should be foregrounded. Furthermore, whilst existing ethical debates about various forms and facets of palliative sedation and, in particular, continuous deep sedation contain important points, it is nevertheless the case that the ethical imperative practicing healthcare professionals involved in end of life care should be most concerned with is the alleviation and management of pain and suffering.

Keywords Palliative care · End of life · Sedation · Symptom control · Suffering · Ethics

12.1 Introduction

Given the extensive literature on the topic it seems clear that palliative sedation raises a particularly challenging set of ethical questions; it is, as van Deldan (2007) has said of terminal sedation, a source of restless debate. Nevertheless, Savulescu

---

N. Emmerich (✉)
Australian National University, Canberra, Australia
e-mail: Nathan.Emmerich@anu.edu.au

P. Mallia et al. (eds.), *Challenges to the Global Issue of End of Life Care*,
Advancing Global Bioethics 17, https://doi.org/10.1007/978-3-030-86386-9_12

and Radcliffe-Richards (2019) have recently claimed that patients not only have a *right* to analgesia and sedation but to unconsciousness.[1] The implication of this suggestion is that healthcare professionals in general, and palliative care specialists in particular, should induce unconsciousness via the use of anesthetics—and not just sedative and analgesia—if and when this is required to alleviate or manage a patient's suffering. Thus, according to these authors, what many take to be a complex ethical debate is in fact a relatively simply matter of a patient's right not to suffer. It is, therefore, a matter of doing whatever will effectively reduce or eliminate such suffering, particularly when it comes to caring for those who are terminally ill and actively dying. Thus, when a patient's symptoms are refractory, when their pain is intractable, rendering them unconscious is, simply, the appropriate clinical response required of any and all healthcare professionals. The use of analgesia, sedation or anesthetic as a response to suffering means that that the patients level of consciousness will be diminished; if and when the level of suffering is such that the clinical response entails reducing consciousness to zero is of no additional ethical significance.

Unsurprisingly, and as has been the case elsewhere (ten Have and Welie 2014; Horn 2018), this approach is presented as something both those for and against euthanasia or Medical Assistance in Dying (MAID) can support (Savulescu and Radcliffe-Richards 2019). Those who argue for euthanasia do so because they think not all suffering can be effectively palliated. Those who argue against it think that ending the lives of patients is not justified by suffering, even at high levels, and even though they recognize suffering's inherent disvalue. However, this kind of palliative response—in which patients are rendered unconscious if their suffering is such that there is no other way to manage it—eliminates suffering without the need to end patient's lives.

Such perspectives remind us that a desire to alleviate or relieve suffering is what motivates the provision of palliative sedation and, one might add, palliative care more generally. As such there is a fundamental ethical imperative behind palliative sedation, one that is consistent with palliative care as a whole. Whilst the desire to do what is right or good cannot guarantee that what one does or how one does it is indeed *ethical*, it is nevertheless the case that those involved in caring for the dying seek to reduce suffering and promote their patients well being, at least insofar as is possible.

Unfortunately, for some of those who are nearing the end of their lives, the scope of what is possible may not be particularly broad. Indeed, it may be limited to the control and management of terminal ailments and the particular symptoms that dying patients commonly experience—such as breathlessness (dyspnea), vomiting, delirium and pain. Such symptoms can become intolerable, intractable and refractory, which is to say they become increasingly difficult to control and manage. As a result, healthcare professionals can find themselves caring for patients whose suffering is clearly agonizing, both for the patient themselves as well as for those

[1] I will have further comments on this notion of a *right* to unconsciousness and what it might entail.

around them, particularly their family members, whilst being able to do very little. In this context, and in the absence of legislation for euthanasia, inducing sedation to the point of unconsciousness may be the only response available to them.

This essay proceeds as follows. First I set out and examine palliative sedation and the various practice that fall within its scope. I then briefly consider various of the ethical concerns that have been expressed in relation to the use of sedation at the end of life before focusing on the particular topic of CDS and the question of providing ANH. This analysis is followed by some concluding remarks and the suggestion that patients have a right to sedation, including to the point of unconsciousness.

12.2 Palliative Sedation: What Is It That We Are Talking About?

Palliative sedation encompasses a range of clinical practices that, for the purposes of alleviating and managing the patient's symptoms, involve providing sedation and analgesia to patients who are reaching the end of their life.[2] As many have pointed out, the terms used in this context are diverse; they often overlap and are continuing to develop (Morita et al. 2001; Cowan and Walsh 2001; Morita et al. 2002; Claessens et al. 2008; Jones 2013a; Taboada 2015). Initially, there seems to have been a range of relatively undifferentiated practices, all of which involved the use of sedation within palliative care. Then, following publication of an article by Enck (1991), the phrase 'terminal sedation' began to be used to discuss the way palliative care professionals sometimes found it necessary to intensify sedation to the point of inducing unconsciousness in order to manage refractory symptoms or intractable pain.

Subsequently, Morita et al. (2002, p. 449) suggested that the phrase 'terminal sedation' was open to misinterpretation. Not only could it be mistaken for the use of sedatives to terminate a patient's life, but the fact that what was being done was an attempt to alleviate or palliate symptoms that were otherwise unmanageable is not made clear. Thus, given neither phrase clearly distinguishes between patients that receive fairly high levels of sedation, but in whom some degree of consciousness can be retained, and those whose symptoms are so intractable and the level of their suffering so great as to result in them needing to be maintained in an unconscious state until death, both 'terminal sedation' and 'palliative sedation'—the phrase preferred by Morita and his co-authors (2001, 2002)—should be taken as overarching labels for a set of practices that require further specification and that can and should be further differentiated.

[2] Whilst it is true to say that the concerns of palliative medicine are greater than end of life care, caring for dying patients does constitute a large part of the field (Emmerich 2018). Furthermore, the kinds of ethical issues that have concerned those who comment upon palliative sedation focus on dying patients. Thus, for the purposes of this paper, palliative care is equated with providing care at the end of life.

One result of such terminological debates is that the phrases 'continuous sedation' and 'continuous deep sedation' (CDS) have subsequently emerged as the preferred, but nevertheless competing, terms for referring to the practice of rendering patients unconscious in response to refractory or intractable symptoms (Sterckx et al. 2013; Morita et al. 2016). More recently Emmerich and Gordijn (2019) have drawn attention to 'crisis sedation', a practice that is usually absent from both clinical and ethical discussions of palliative and terminal sedation. Thus, despite the fact that there is a fairly expansive literature dedicated to debating these phrases and the range of practices they represent, no entirely clear, precise or definitive terminology has resulted. Furthermore, it seems no exact terms will be found. As such Jones, for example, presents terminal sedation as a label for "a large set of possible practices each with its own ethical significance, some being acceptable forms of palliative care, some being forms of euthanasia, and some fitting into neither category" (Jones 2013b, p. 63).[3] Such conceptual debates might be taken to reflect a certain and, one might add, *inherent* level of imprecision within the practice of sedation in palliative care. In the active management of dying patients the art of medicine comes to the fore. The meaning of palliative sedation is, then, marked by certain degree of ambiguity and uncertainty, at least insofar as it names a number of more or less well-differentiated practices.

12.3 Ethics and Palliative Sedation

Whilst the concern existed prior to the advent of palliative care and, therefore, to the clinical introduction of palliative sedation, the primary ethical issue associated with this type of care has been the question of hastening death.[4] However, whilst it is commonly thought that providing sedation risks hastening the moment of death, recent research has disputed this presumption (Mercadante et al. 2009; Maltoni et al. 2009, 2012). Furthermore, as a central part of palliative care, it would seem that the appropriate use of palliative sedation has the potential to extend life as well as alleviate suffering, thereby promoting patient's quality of life. The use of palliative sedation can, therefore, be considered as ethical imperative and something bioethicists ought to advocate for, particularly when one considers the fact that pain has tended to go undertreated (Rich 1997).

Whilst concerns about hastening death through the use of sedatives and analgesia may be unwarranted when a patient is being cared for in relatively ideal circumstances and in the context of relatively advanced palliative care services, this may

[3] Whether or not euthanasia or MAID falls within the bounds of palliative and / or terminal sedation is, like much else in this area, controversial. Whilst one can see both sides of the issue, given that we will not be considering any action that has the patient's death as its aim in this chap. I will not be adopting a definitive position.

[4] Of course, the issue of hastening death is closely aligned with questions about causing death, but this latter concern is beyond the scope of this chapter.

not always be the case. Thus, concerns about hastening death may well be an issue for those practicing in more challenging contexts. Such contexts may include caring for patients who wish to die at home with a minimal level of intervention by healthcare professionals as well as cases where informal caregivers are involved in managing medications. More obviously it applies to the developing world and to countries where palliative care services are under developed or resourced. Nevertheless, here the traditional appeal to the Doctrine of Double Effect can be made. It is not unethical to risk hastening death as long as ones actions do not aim at this end, but at some other ethical purpose that would otherwise be unobtainable.

It is, then, licit to risk hastening death as long as this risk is merely a foreseen side effect of a treatment that is motivated by an ethical imperative, such as the relief of suffering, that cannot be achieved by other means. That this ethical principle has been improperly realized by many healthcare professionals has, arguable, made a significant contribution to the under treatment of the pain and suffering experienced by dying patients. Whilst the realties of clinical practice may complicate the principle, particularly when it comes to discerning what we intend and what we merely foresee it nevertheless provides a basis on which we can begin to perceive the risk of hastening death as something that should be balanced with the risk of allowing pain and suffering to go untreated.

Whilst the focus on pain and suffering—or its alleviation and management—is not (or should not be) unique to palliative care it is nevertheless the case that it is the primary focus of the specialty. At this juncture it is worth saying something about the nature of pain and, especially, suffering, both in general and in the context of the end of life. As Rich points out, the alleviation of suffering should be a cardinal principle of medical ethics and practice. However, we should note that it is simplistic to associate suffering with pain as a physiological phenomenon and physical or bodily sensation or experience. Rather, it is the case that "[s]uffering is an affliction of persons, not bodies" (Cassell and Rich 2010, p. 436). Furthermore, according to Cassell:

> Suffering occurs when an impending destruction of the person is perceived; it continues until the threat of disintegration has passed or until the integrity of the person can be restored in some other manner. … [S]uffering extends beyond the physical. Most generally, suffering can be defined as the state of severe distress associated with events that threaten the intactness of person[s]. (Cassell 2003, p. 32)

When Cassell speaks of the intactness of persons he is not merely referring to some biological threat, and its physiological consequences for the patients body. Rather, as a phenomenologist, he is concerned with the intactness of our *selves* as embodied beings. Given this view, it is unavoidably the case that threats to our biological or bodily existence also represent threats to our existence as conscious and self-aware beings. Our embodied nature is such that, although we can contemplate the Cartesian distinction between body and mind, our internal experience of self cannot practically maintain or *inhabit* the dualist position. As a result, whilst we can reflect upon our mortality and the impermanence of both our bodies as well as our existential existence in the abstract this differs significantly from actually experiencing a particular illness, particularly one that represents some kind of existential threat (Carel 2008).

Such threats may vary. They may, for example, be acute and appreciably related to our mortality, as in the case of receiving a cancer diagnosis or a heart attack[5]; they may also be relatively minimal and highly likely to be transient, as when one has the flu or a broken arm; or they may be chronic and debilitating, as is the case for those living with neurodegenerative disorders or Lymphangioleiomyomatosis (LAM).[6] In each case the vulnerability of our existence is exposed and, as a result, there is the potential for suffering, and for there to be some embodied experience of vulnerability and distress related to the intactness of the person. Cassell's account is such that patients who are suffering are not, simply, minds having or experiencing certain kinds of bodily sensations. The nature of suffering is that, by exposing the vulnerability of our existence, it affects our minds, the way we are, and even who we are or, to put it another way, who it is that we can be.

This is particularly pertinent as a diminished level of consciousness can be the consequence of providing patients with sedatives and/ or analgesia, and some medical professionals can be reluctant to risk this side effect. However, once we realise that the nature of suffering is such that it can impact our consciousness and, albeit in a different sort of way, can diminish it, the concerns motivating such reluctance seem to be of less significance. Patients who are suffering are often withdrawn and find interacting with others difficult and even undesirable. This is, of course, entirely comprehensible when we reflect on how we feel when we are vulnerable. Patients who are dying, and whose suffering is particularly acute, may also experience confusion and even delirium. In this context it would seem clear that an appropriate balance needs to be struck between the impact of sedative and analgesia on the patient's consciousness, the appropriate management of symptoms, and the broader consequences of suffering.

Furthermore, one should also bear in mind that the debilitating effects of suffering are likely to be cumulative, particularly in patients who are dying. Such patients are declining towards death, the stresses and strains experienced in the earlier parts of this process may have consequences in the later stages. In this view, providing optimal palliative care and sedation is not simply about the present moment, but about the bigger picture: the trajectory of the patient and their illness as a whole. Thus, palliative sedation does not appear to negatively impact survival times of dying patients (Maltoni et al. 2012). Indeed, many argue that the earlier palliative care specialists become involved in the care of patients with terminal illnesses the better (Rowland and Schumann 2010). Thus, the proper use of palliative care does not simply alleviate suffering in the present, nor it its concern limited to the patients broader quality of life, it can also be represented as contributing to longevity.

---

[5] At this point it is worth referencing the notion of an existential slap, something that can form part of the patient's experience when being given a terminal diagnosis (Coyle 2004).

[6] The example is chosen as the philosopher Havi Carel (2008) has written about her experiences of having LAM and theorized the nature of illness on this basis.

12.4 Palliative Sedation, Nutrition and Hydration

When providing care at the end of life managing a patient's nutrition and hydration is often an issue for healthcare professionals. Given food and water are commonly understood as being universal basic needs that no one should be without, discussing whether or not fluids and nutrition should be provided often perceived as being loaded or biased in some way. Seen in this light, it seems as if some perceive withdrawing food and intravenous fluids as, in effect, an attempt to hasten death by definition. This is, however, a mistaken perception. Both nutrition and hydration can become clinically burdensome to patients and, in some circumstances, continuing to provide them can increase suffering and negatively impact both the patient's quality of life and its remaining length.

In the context of palliative sedation questions concerning withdrawing or withholding nutrition and hydration have contributed to the perception that some practices, notable that of Continuous Deep Sedation, amount to 'slow euthanasia.' The suggestion cuts both ways. Those who are concerned about the morality of euthanasia and assisted dying worry that CDS is the thin end of the wedge, whilst those who think euthanasia or assisted dying should be provided in some form may consider CDS to be a fudge. The fact that CDS has apparently been used to avoid broader discussion of euthanasia and assisted dying may compound these concerns (Horn 2018). However, pace my previous argument, it would seem that if the provision of sedation, including sedation to the point of unconsciousness, should be based on an evaluation of the patient's clinical status then one might also suggest the same of Artificial Nutrition and Hydration (ANH), both in general and in the particular case of end of life care.

To recap, given the physiological control healthcare professionals can exercise through the use of opiates, sedatives and even anesthesia, it would seem clearly unethical for patients and, in particular, dying patients to be allowed to suffer needlessly. Of course this is something that patients themselves may express divergent views upon; they may vary in the levels of suffering they are willing to experience or endure. Thus, an open discussion of the potential of sedative, opiates and anesthesia to manage pain coupled with their likely effect on the patient's level of consciousness seems warranted. As a result, whilst remaining within the boundaries of clinical guidelines as well as the patient's wishes, preferences and decisions, there seems clear ethical warrant for the provision of sedation. Where necessary, this includes sedating patients to the point of inducing (and permanently maintaining) unconsciousness as well as when encountering the possibility it will hasten death.

It seems to me that one might evaluate the provision of ANH in a similar manner, i.e. with regard to the suffering of patients and whether or not it will be alleviated or exacerbated. Certainly, the existing motivation for withdrawing or withholding ANH from patients relates to the fact that it can be a burdensome for patients. Whilst the need for food and fluids is rightly seen as a basic requirement for biological life, that does not indicate that dying human organisms necessarily benefit from being provided with intravenous food and fluids when they can no longer tolerate them orally. Not only might they put greater strain on the patient's body, but their provision may also necessitate repeated attempts to insert and reinsert IV lines. Furthermore, once in place, they might restrict the patient's movements or simply become an unnecessary nuisance.

This is not, of course, to say that dying patients who wish to eat or drink should not be allowed to do so. Even if a decision has been made not to implement ANH it would seem good practice to ensure dying patients always have access to fresh water and ice chips. Furthermore, even if a patient is disinclined to consume fluids orally, a moistened sponge can nevertheless be used to refresh their mouths. The non-provision of ANH does not, as some in the British media supposed during the largely manufactured furor over the Liverpool Care Pathway (McCartney 2012; Wrigley 2014), condemn patients to die in a state of starvation or dehydration. Rather, it recognizes that neither fluids nor nutrition necessarily alleviate suffering in all cases and circumstances. Furthermore, as both hunger and thirst can wane towards the end of life, their absence does not necessarily result in further suffering.

In this context it would seem that decisions about providing ANH to dying patients, including those who are receiving palliative sedation, are not necessarily ethical questions. Or, at least, they should not be treated as ethical questions first and foremost. Rather, the (non)provision of ANH should primarily be seen as a clinical matter; a question of what the best course of care and treatment for this patient might be. In short, we should ask ourselves whether or not ANH represents a benefit or a burden to the patient. Furthermore, rather than focus on longevity alone, we should be concerned with the patient's suffering. Thus, even if fluids are likely to benefit a patient insofar as it will likely postpone death a short while, one should consider the burdens their provision might present; will providing IV fluids increase or decrease the burden of suffering experienced by the patient? Will cause or prevent further suffering? (cf Craig 2005 and associated commentaries) This is, of course, different to considering the suffering that might result from a prolonged death or period of dying.

Whilst it may seem that I am arguing that should be decided in ethical terms as concerns, one should recall that if ANH causes suffering it does so by placing strain on the patients body and its biological systems, at least in part. If ANH is likely to be a source of suffering then it is unlikely to prolong the patient life. Thus, at least to some degree, the ethical concerns one might have over decisions regarding the non-provision of ANH to dying patients are reflected in the clinical picture, and the decisions we might make in its light. The mistake comes when ethical concerns are allowed to overtake the clinical realities healthcare professionals are faced with. Whilst medicine and palliative care have an underlying and broad moral motivation, this then needs to be accounted for in the light of proper clinical assessment of both individual cases and the more general insights derived from biomedical research and embedded in professional guidelines (and pathways). Medical ethics, and those who offer commentaries on the topic, need to be responsive to the facts, the realities inhabited by terminally ill and suffering patients and those seeking to care for them.

Before moving on, however, we should take the time to reflect on ANH in the context of CDS. Arguably, if a patient is sedated to the point on unconsciousness and the intention is to maintain them in this state, then there would not appear to be any reason to act so as to prolong their life. However, the effect of this would be to provide significant support to those who perceive CDS as 'slow euthanasia'. Thus, one might instead respond by supposing that since CDS patients are beyond the point of any further suffering, providing ANH cannot present a further burden and so should be continued, if only to militate against comparing euthanasia with CDS and the withdrawal of ANH (Holm 2013). Whilst this may be correct, it is incorrect to presume that ANH necessarily prolongs the life of dying patients; it may in fact hasten it in some cases. As such, it seems better to predicate the provision of ANH in unconscious patients on the way in which one would treat a clinically equivalent patient who is not being maintained in an unconscious state.

12.5 Conclusion

In this chapter I have suggested that an over abundance of ethical caution may be an inhibiting factor when it comes to the provision of sedation to dying patients. Furthermore, this is arguably compounded when it comes to the intricacy of the debate in relation to CDS and the provision of ANH, not least due to the phrase 'slow euthanasia.' My response has been to suggest that those involved in palliative care and the sedation of dying patients should be led by the imperative to alleviate suffering and, as a result, give priority to their clinical judgment and the underlying moral motivation of palliative care and medicine as a whole. Of course, this should take place in the context of best practice guidelines as well as open communication with the patient and, where appropriate, their families.

Given this stance we might review the notion of a right to be unconscious, as proposed by Savulescu and Radcliffe-Richards (2019) or to CDS, as per recent French legislation (Horn 2018). Such a right could be understood in a variety of ways. First, it might mean nothing more than sedation being available in a particular set of circumstances. If, say, I have a right to speak to my constituency MP, this can be met by the fact that they have a surgery once a month. It does not mean I have a right to speak to them whenever I wish to do so, using their personal telephone number. Nor does it mean I have a right to demand they speak with me at a time and place of my choosing. One can think similarly when it comes to a right to unconsciousness. The suggestion is not that one can demand unconsciousness as and when one wishes to do so, the right only obtains in particular sets of circumstances. The question then becomes one of who gets to decide when those circumstances have obtained. This is, of course, primarily a matter of clinical judgment and, furthermore, something that may well only emerge in the context of treating or *caring for* the patient over time. One should not resort to CDS before attempting to meet the patient's needs without rendering them unconscious.

It seems, then, that a right to be unconscious does not or should not be taken to mean that patients can demand CDS or similar. The proposal would seem to be, then, that clinicians should be both able and prepared to provide this level of care if and when the needs of the patient dictate it should be provided. Calling for, or instituting, such rights would seem somewhat misguided or a way to avoid dealing with bigger or more intractable issues. In France this would seem to be an intransigent medical culture that has not kept pace with advances in palliative care. Whilst introducing a right to CDS may be politically strategic, whether or not it does much for actual patients remains to be seen.

One can think similarly with regard Savulescu and Radcliffe-Richards proposals. Indeed, it is more difficult to see what grounds or motivates the right, other than the more general notion that patients should receive the medical care they need. In this context it would seem better to promote the development of palliative care protocols that encompass and delimit the practice of CDS. It would also seem better to advocate for the further development of palliative care services and to ensure that they are accessible to all those who need them. Indeed, one might even worry about the unintended consequences of introducing a right to CDS or to be unconscious might have. A focus on this kind of sedation may have a detrimental impact of developing services to provide sedation at lower levels, including both hospices and services for patients who wish to remain at home. Attempting to ensure patients receive the proper level of pain relief might be one way to understand the right to unconsciousness proposed by Savulescu and Radcliffe-Richards. Nevertheless, there would seem to be other ways to promote the same goal and to do so more effectively. It is the latter that we should most vigorously pursue.

Bibliography

Carel, H. 2008. *Illness*. Acumen Publishing.

Cassell, E.J. 2003. *The nature of suffering and the goals of medicine*. Oxford, UK: Oxford University Press.

Cassell, E.J., and B.A. Rich. 2010. Intractable end-of-life suffering and the ethics of palliative sedation. *Pain Medicine* 11: 435–438. https://doi.org/10.1111/j.1526-4637.2009.00786.x.

Claessens, P., J. Menten, P. Schotsmans, and B. Broeckaert. 2008. Palliative sedation: A review of the research literature. *Journal of Pain and Symptom Management* 36: 310–333.

Cowan, J.D., and D. Walsh. 2001. Terminal sedation in palliative medicine—definition and review of the literature. *Support Care Cancer* 9: 403–407.

Coyle, N. 2004. The existential slap—A crisis of disclosure. *International Journal of Palliative Nursing* 10: 520. https://doi.org/10.12968/ijpn.2004.10.11.17130.

Craig, G. 2005. Sedation without hydration can seriously damage your health. *International Journal of Palliative Nursing* 11: 333–337. https://doi.org/10.12968/ijpn.2005.11.7.18485.

Emmerich, N. 2018. Leadership in palliative medicine: Moral, ethical and educational. *BMC Medical Ethics* 19: 55. https://doi.org/10.1186/s12910-018-0296-z.

Emmerich, N., and B. Gordijn. 2019. Ethics of crisis sedation: Questions of performance and consent. *Journal of Medical Ethics medethics-2018-105285*. https://doi.org/10.1136/medethics-2018-105285.

Enck, R.E. 1991. Drug-induced terminal sedation for symptom control. *The American Journal of Hospice & Palliative Care* 8: 3–5.

Holm, S. 2013. 14 – terminal sedation and euthanasia: The virtue in calling a spade what it is. In *Continuous sedation at the end of life: Ethical, clinical and legal perspectives*, ed. S. Sterckx, K. Raus, and F. Mortier. Cambridge, UK: Cambridge University Press.

Horn, R. 2018. The 'French exception': The right to continuous deep sedation at the end of life. *Journal of Medical Ethics* 44: 204–205. https://doi.org/10.1136/medethics-2017-104484.

Jones, D.A. 2013a. Death by equivocation: A manifold definition of terminal sedation. In *Continuous sedation at the end of life: Ethical, clinical and legal perspectives*, ed. S. Sterckx, K. Raus, and F. Mortier. Cambridge, UK: Cambridge University Press.

———. 2013b. 3 – Death by equivocation: A manifold definition of terminal sedation. In *Continuous sedation at the end of life: Ethical, clinical and legal perspectives*, ed. S. Sterckx, K. Raus, and F. Mortier. Cambridge, UK: Cambridge University Press.

Maltoni, M., C. Pittureri, E. Scarpi, et al. 2009. Palliative sedation therapy does not hasten death: Results from a prospective multicenter study. *Annals of Oncology* 20: 1163–1169. https://doi.org/10.1093/annonc/mdp048.

Maltoni, M., E. Scarpi, M. Rosati, et al. 2012. Palliative sedation in end-of-life care and survival: A systematic review. *JCO* 30: 1378–1383. https://doi.org/10.1200/JCO.2011.37.3795.

McCartney, M. 2012. The assault on the Liverpool care pathway. *BMJ* 345: e7316–e7316. https://doi.org/10.1136/bmj.e7316.

Mercadante, S., G. Intravaia, P. Villari, et al. 2009. Controlled sedation for refractory symptoms in dying patients. *Journal of Pain and Symptom Management* 37: 771–779. https://doi.org/10.1016/j.jpainsymman.2008.04.020.

Morita, T., I. Maeda, M. Mori, et al. 2016. Uniform definition of continuous-deep sedation. *Lancet Oncology* 17: e222.

Morita, T., S. Tsuneto, and Y. Shima. 2001. Proposed definitions for terminal sedation. *Lancet* 358: 335–336. https://doi.org/10.1016/S0140-6736(01)05515-5.

———. 2002. Definition of sedation for symptom relief: A systematic literature review and a proposal of operational criteria. *Journal of Pain and Symptom Management* 24: 447–453.

Rich, B.A. 1997. A legacy of silence: Bioethics and the culture of pain. *Journal of Medical Humanities* 18: 233–259. https://doi.org/10.1023/A:1025697920944.

Rowland, K., and S.-A. Schumann. 2010. Palliative care: Earlier is better. *The Journal of Family Practice* 59: 695–698.

Savulescu, J., and J. Radcliffe-Richards. 2019. A right to be unconscious. *Anaesthesia*. https://doi.org/10.1111/anae.14635.

Sterckx, S., K. Raus, and F. Mortier, eds. 2013. *Continuous sedation at the end of life: Ethical, clinical and legal perspectives*. Cambridge University Press.

Taboada, P. 2015. Sedation at the end of life. Clinical realities, trends and current debate. In *Sedation at the end-of-life: An interdisciplinary approach*, 1–14. Dordrecht: Springer.

ten Have, H., and J.V. Welie. 2014. Palliative sedation versus euthanasia: An ethical assessment. *Journal of Pain and Symptom Management* 47: 123–136.

van Delden, J.J.M. 2007. Terminal sedation: Source of a restless ethical debate. *Journal of Medical Ethics* 33: 187–188. https://doi.org/10.1136/jme.2007.020446.

Wrigley, A. 2014. Ethics and end of life care: The Liverpool care pathway and the Neuberger review. *Journal of Medical Ethics Medethics-2013-101780*. https://doi.org/10.1136/medethics-2013-101780.

Part IV
Implementing-Change Pathways

Chapter 13
Engaging Patient Groups in End-of-Life

Gertrude Buttigieg and Christopher Vella

Abstract Patient organisations on a local and national level offer an important insight in the area in which they operate. They are made of people who are in direct contact with the situation of a disease or condition but also know the cultural realities, religious beliefs and customs of the people. End-of-life issues are closely linked to the culture and respective nature of the condition or the experience of each person. Like other areas of healthcare patient organisations promote dignity in care and giving patients a voice at such a delicate stage in life. Through a discussion, highlights of possible models are explored based on patient empowerment to give patient an active role, together with his/her carers to express and seek what he/she considers to be the best options for him or her. It is a very diverse argument when considering the global perspective however the patients' organisations can help patients directly as well as help formulation of services and policies relating to end-of-life care.

Keywords Patients' groups · Organisations · Empowerment · Education · Experience

13.1 Patient Organisations

Need and personal experience often leads to people to get together and slowly get to form a support group. These groups have developed over the years and have become more organized and regulated. There are varies laws in different countries to regulate these entities. According to the International Alliance of Patients Organisations (IAPO) (www.iapo.org.uk) '*Patients' Organisations are important patient advocates that truly understand patients' needs*'. These organisations are usually non-governmental patient organisations, set up not-for-profit as patient representative groups. The structures and remit of these organisations is also considerably diverse.

G. Buttigieg (✉) · C. Vella (✉)
Malta Health Network, Marsa, Malta

P. Mallia et al. (eds.), *Challenges to the Global Issue of End of Life Care*,
Advancing Global Bioethics 17, https://doi.org/10.1007/978-3-030-86386-9_13

Some groups operate as local patients' organisations – these often deal with single conditions or diseases and unite to give a stronger voice than a single individual. The people within these organisations, their administration and regulatory structures make a big difference of how well and effective these organisations become. Local patients' organisations are often established in a specific city, town or district within a defined geographic area. Being together helps the patients to share experiences however in small rural areas these organisations may find it difficult to operate and thus in some countries people have found that national organisations a better means of setting up. This often works out well to avoid duplication of work and educational campaigns or support offered and are more cost effective. National patients' organisations bring together groups of patients at a country level. National organisations may be disease specific or they may bring together various smaller groups working across different disease or conditions often referred to as umbrella organisations. Again the organisation at national level of these varies between countries, since in some places there are logistical even language barriers within the same country. In return the National organisations may seek affiliation or collaboration within bigger groups on Regional or International Level. Again these may be condition specific or bring together different groups. Such an example on a regional level are the European Association of Palliative care(EAPC) (https://www.eapcnet.eu/home). EAPC brings together associations from 33 European countries. It's members focus specifically on perspectives related to palliative care. On the other hand there are non-specific conditions, such as the European Patients' Forum (EPF) (http://www.eu-patient.eu/). EPF brings together over 70 members which are pan-European disease specific patients' organisations and national coalition platforms of patients' organisations from different issues but coming from the same country. On a higher level one finds International patients' organisations, these represent groups of patients at a worldwide level such as IAPO which is an umbrella patients' organization which brings together tens of organisations from all over the World and different areas of interest or disease and conditions. International organisations exist also on for specific conditions such as International Association for Hospice and Palliative care (IAHPC) (https://hospicecare.com) which links one to global organisations which support people needing palliative care around the World. Through their Global Directory of Palliative Care one can find there relevant organisation which deals with palliative care in every corner of the Globe.

Patient organisations on a local and national level offer an important insight in the area in which they operate. They are made of people who are in direct contact with the situation of a disease or condition but also know the cultural realities, religious beliefs and customs of the people. End-of-life issues are closely linked to the culture and respective nature of the condition or the experience of each person. The person's views towards death and process leading to death, varies between cultures. Whilst in most developed countries support and literature about end-of-life and palliative services are mostly focused towards terminally cancer patients in less developed countries such as sub-Saharan Africa the bigger concern is HIV/AIDS (Gysels et al. 2011) whilst in areas where longevity and an ageing population is on the increase the needs for these patients vary immensely. For many people what used to be considered as a 'terminally ill' a matter of months this may now turn into years leading to life with more extended chronic conditions rather than the typically way one considers a terminal illness (Zaman et al. 2017).

End-of-life care over the years has become very controversial. The fine line between medical care, improving medical technologies and therapies and the quality of life of the individual are often very difficult to delineate. Zaman et al. (2017) describe the shift in beliefs around dying from a religious belief to a medical process. The complex dynamics between the needs of the persons and the heavy burden for families and caregivers also merits to be highlighted at this point. The tri-partite view of patient, carers and medics is very much a matter of great interest and at heart of patient organisations. In fact the goal of Hospice care is primarily that of helping people who are dying to die in peace, comfort and dignity (Lu et al. 2018). Again the meaning of dignity at the end-of-life opens up to various dimensions, which have a different definition for patient, carer and professionals. However all seem to agree about the dimensions of suffering and the need to help the patients to a varying degree – physical – including pain management, social, psychological and spiritual. Patient organisations of various chronic conditions such as heart conditions, cancer, HIV/AIDS etc. are usually the first point of contact for these patients even before these patients have to face the fact that 'life-is-short'. Whilst in 'Hospice' terms usually palliative refers to the last 6 months in the life of a person, the accuracy of how long or short this term can be may vary. Thus the role of the patient organisations in touch with the patient even prior to this stage is considered very important. Palliative care is to be considered as a process whereby the trust relationship between patient, carers and professional team assists the person to this journey marked by the inevitable truth of letting death take its course. The *Quebec End-of-Life Palliative Care Policy (2004)*uses a term which I find very important in our discussion '*The need to be well informed and supported when making a decision*' (pg 18).

13.2 Patient Empowerment

The World Health Organisation (WHO) (2009) defines empowerment as "*a process through which people gain greater control over decisions and actions affecting their health*" (WHO 2009, pg.190). Off course at this stage of discussion about end-of-life decisions this concept certainly applies. This should be seen as both an individual and community process. Patient empowerment is not a one-way process. Empowerment of citizens and patients is a task which involves and encourages interaction of communities, health care professionals, policy makers and all other civil society actors with respect to health and well being of individuals. This is a process of the patient from a passive recipient of care to an active partner in their health care and decision making process. Both IAPO and EPF have published valuable documentation speaking about the importance of patient empowerment and how patient organisations have a crucial role in this. Patient empowerment is defined in multiple ways depending on the context and objectives. EPF (2015a, b) defines it as a "*process that helps people gain control over their own lives and increases their capacity to act on issues that they themselves define as important*" (EPF 2015a, b, pg 4). Aspects of empowerment include health literacy, shared decision-making and self-management (EPF 2015a, b). EPF has produced various literature including a toolkit (EPF 2017) which is a very valuable tool for patients, professionals and organisations. The principles which emerge from patient empowerment are the Five 'E''s: Education, Experience, Expertise, Equality and Engagement (EPF 2015a, b, 2).

Education Whenever a patient receives a diagnosis, especially one which does not have a veryfavourable prognosis, the patient will need some time before adjusting to this new reality. Once the initial shock has faded, this person will invariably need to know as much as he/she can in order to be able to make their individual decisions. For patients to be able to make informed decisions about their health, they need to be able to access all the relevant information, in an easily understandable format. The first step, and most crucial one, is the ability of the patient to distinguish between sources. Having a relationship between professionals and patient organisations built on mutual respect, and towards achievement of a common goal, means that correctly suggesting relevant patients' organizations ensure that the information obtained is from a reliable and verified source.

WHO, 2014 estimated that annually worldwide 377 per 100,000 adult population over the age of 15 and 63 out of 100,000 under 15-year olds required palliative care at the end-of-life. These numbers are clearly millions when translated into world population. This further highlights the diversity of situations when one is looking at support and decisions needed at end-of-life globally. The causes of death also vary between regions in the World whilst what WHO (2014) also clearly outlines is the discrepancies and again the needs of approximately 1.2 million children who require palliative care world-wide is considerable. Patient and Charitable organisations operating within an area or a specialized patient group are placed in the better position know the culture, beliefs and the strengths and weakness within that group. Zaman et al. (2017) argue that despite the fact that dying is a universal human experience a global approach to end-of-life issues is not practical. They stress that one needs to take into account the multiple features in the care of the dying even within-country variations and diversity of provision. They end their argument by recommending that effective ways of dealing with end-of-life issues must be culturally appropriate and the sustainability depends on their particularity rather than on the universality. Organisations operating at a local level are the best placed entities to interact with the locals since they are familiar with the resources and services available. These organisations can reach out with education programmes and resources within the community they operate. Whilst at a day and age of technology and everything happening online and in social media, one has to keep in mind that the realities of illiteracy, poor health literacy, poor digital literacy and poor access to what some would consider the basic of basic still exists. Patient organisations would know of these realities and are best placed to reach the patients most in need. An example quoted by WHO (2014) is the St. Giles Hospice which is an independent voluntary sector organization offering specialist palliative care services in a mixed professional-volunteer model as indicated by the ratio of approximately 240 paid staff to 1200 volunteers. This Hospice operates like others in the UK where they focus on engaging with local communities. These Hospices run health promotion and well being programmes as well as supportive social care. Their programmes not only focus on end-of-life care but support carers and resilience being in the community. They work with schools and prisons whilst running bereavement support services. These services are supported by professional services which intervene in the severe of cases.

WHO, 2015 recognised that education material for patients and carers can be made available in various ways '*including information leaflets, online peer support, one-to-one counselling, group education sessions, telephone coaching, technology to monitor symptoms, and psychological behaviour change interventions*' WHO 2015 (pg. 3). The same document stresses the importance of '*interventions which are co-created and co-led by service users and professionals more often result in positive outcomes*' WHO, 2015 (pg. 3). Although the WHO, 2015 directs the argument about self-management the same arguments are equally valid when looking at end-of-life issues including matters such as advance care planning. This is the process whereby one makes his/her wishes know in advance about personal and financial matters should they be in a position where they are unable to make a decision for themselves.

Mallia et al. (2017) explain that Advance Care plan is not an officially signed legal document like Advance Directive but is more focused on management of patient care at a time when the patient is still considered in a capable frame of mind to take and express his/her decisions, in line with recognized legal parameters in the respective country. Patients' organisations are well placed to provide appropriate information and education and thus assisting patients and carers to plan adequately and take share responsibility in their decisions. These may include the choice of carers, the choice of place of care and the degree of interventions should the need arise, the pain management options available etc. Information packs are often prepared by organisations such as Hospices working in certain regions or areas. These packs have valuable information such as what services are available for the persons in the area, what one can do at home and what to expect. Another example of best-practice offered by a patient organisation is the initiative of Caring Community (USA) (www.caringcommunity.org) which provides a support checklist available in English and Spanish and looks at a holistic approach to end-of-life issues which may vary in importance between patient and professionals. Areas looked into include personal values such as quality of life, preferred logistics for care, advanced directives, familial communication and a other considerations such as spiritual and after death arrangements. Similar tools are made available by the Marie Curie Foundation (www.mariecurie.org.uk). Interesting information is also available for care givers. Such an example are the brochures and online resources made available by the Victoria Hospice, British Columbia e.g. Preparing for Death – A Guide for Caregivers and other advice for the person facing a terminal illness. The information is presented in an easy manner and whilst the person is encouraged to face the reality of the situation the person is given practical advice with a telephone number where one can access volunteers to speak to at such delicate situations. On the other hand the information to caregivers outlines practical ways of how a patient can react, what to expect and how to take care of the patient and oneself since caring for a terminally-ill patient may be very burdensome physically and emotionally. However knowing that there is support readily available at a phone call away makes all the difference for both patient and carer. In fact these resources often facilitate the person's wish to die at home.

Timely training and support on self-management is important at different points of the health continuum by individuals that seek to maintain good health and prevent illnesses and by patients living with long-term conditions. Several online training and resources are available for patients, carers and patient advocates, provided by patients' organisations through various projects. Two such projects worth mentioning, although they are European initiatives, being online tools they are accessed worldwide these are, the European Patients' Advocacy Programme (EPAP) and European Patients' Academy for Therapeutic Innovation (EUPATI). EPAP is a self-learning programme introducing patients and carers to the essential skills and knowledge needed to interact with healthcare professionals, policy makers, researchers and journalists. It was developed by the European Lung Foundation, (ELF) with active contributions of patients and professionals with expertise in key areas. The course covers 8 modules all offered online and a certificate is obtained at the end of each module. The 8 modules are Becoming better informed, Improving public awareness, Improving treatment and care, Supporting research and development, Influencing policy, Working with the media, Participating in Health Care Conferences and International Health Research Project. The programme is in English language but the site offers resources in Dutch too. An interesting multilingual site is that provided by the EUPATI. EUPATI was the result of the fast advancing scenario of medicines development which required active participation of patients. However unless patients were given the required information they were not actively participating. Also there is a paradigm shift of patients being considered as partners and thus this required more trained patients and patient advocates. EUPATI which started in 2012 is now offering Patient Expert training courses which are a combination of online self-learning, 2 face-to-face events and a patient involvement forum and a rich website full of resources which is available in 9 languages including Danish, English, French, German, Italian, Dutch, Polish, Russian and Spanish. Although the primary emphasis of EUPATI was the development of medicines, the site offers reliable medical information which is useful for every patient, carer, patient advocate and professionals alike.

Experience Individual patients work with patient organisations to represent them, channeling their experiences and their voices into a unified cry for improvement. The experience is closely linked to the beliefs and cultures. The conceptions about death, death anxiety, bereavement, and burial ritualsare different across cultures. Thus before looking at the individual patients one needs to take into account where they are coming from, what is culturally and socio-economically appropriate and acceptable for them. The importance of spirituality has an important role in an end-of-life care, which affects directly the quality of life, quality of care and overall health and well being of patients (Winkelman et al. 2011; Astrow et al. 2018; Bai and Lazenby 2015). Whilst individual professionals, institutions or a charitable entity may have the best intensions for setting up services and providing support for end-of-life patients however if they do not understand the culture in which they are operating they are doomed to fail from go. Time constraints and unpreparedness are the two most cited factors which limit inputs from the individual professionals (Balboni et al. 2014; Phelps et al. 2012). Gire (2014) gives an extensive discussion on the cultural influence on the concept of death and dying. Religious and cultural traditions certainly have an impact on one's views towards death, whilst in Hinduism – life and death are considered a circular continuity one of the other and back again into a new identity, Christians believe that life as we know it occurs only once. Death is a transformation from an earthly body to a spiritual form. In other beliefs such as Buddhism and some Native American tribes to coexistence between dead and living is believed. Whilst in some cultures the dead are kept 'alive' by their beloved ones through memories and memorials in other cultures death signals the end and people are even prohibited from even mentioning the names of the dead. The fact that death is a reality for every person at some point in life is a fact one learns about almost at the moment of birth. Despite this truth to a varying degree people may live with a degree of death anxiety. Gire (2014) explored the death anxiety as related to cultural as well as religious beliefs. Death anxiety seems to be more associated with the psychological wellbeing especially among the elderly, although the degrees to which this impacts the person varies considerably on the culture. Thus when one is planning training or intervention programmes looking at end-of-life services, one needs to be familiar and take into consideration the cultural and religious beliefs in their work. Quoting Gire (2014, pg 10) '*This also underscores the point that there are likely no (or at the most very few) culture-free prescriptions of dealing with death anxiety. Therefore, counselors, social workers, and other practitioners must show extreme sensitivity to, and consider cultural or societal variables operating in the populations they serve, to enhance the likelihood of providing effective interventions.*' Ilemona Ekore and Lanre-Abass (2016) highlight the complexity of views towards death and African cultures leading one to stress the fact that what applies in one culture does not necessarily translate in another. Various patients' organisations based in Africa are a reflection of this where they support families and offer cultural sensitive support to their respective patient group, primarily examples of organisations helping patients and their families include the Community Health and Information Network (CHAIN) http://www.chainproject.co.ug/ which is based in Uganda. CHAIN promotes the empowerment of people living with and affected by HIV&AIDS, tuberculosis (TB), malaria and non-communicable diseases (NCDs). It offers capacity building to community based organisations, supports orphans and vulnerable children (OVC) and their households, youth, women, most at risk populations and other vulnerable people in the community. Similarly Sharecare Ghana (Sharecare4u) http://www.sharecare4u.org is based in Ghana and through its site it reaches out to patients with rare neuroimmunological diseases, autoimmune conditions such as Transverse Myelitis, Acute Disseminated Encephalomyelitis (ADEM), Neuromyelitis Optica (Devic's disease), Rheumatoid Arthritis, Multiple Sclerosis, Lupus and neurological diseases, their families, carers and friends or important others. It offers the opportunity to patients and their carers opportunities to explore treatment options, discuss their expectations, share their experience or simply offer a listening ear. A similar organisation assisting AIDS patients in Uganda is The Aids Support Organisation http://www.tasouganda.org.

These are real examples that patient organisations can offer so much when they use their native cultural experience coupled with disease/condition experience.

The carer experience is worth looking at, at this stage. It is true that most of the focus is often put on the patient. However during the course of an illness, especially a terminal illness the role of the carer is very crucial. The matter of care at home versus care at hospital is a very important argument. Again the role of culture and family dynamics plays a big role. In the African cultures, where the role of the extended family and where hospital facilities are very lacking, the role of the carers is very crucial. Ilemona Ekore and Lanre-Abass (2016) explains the dynamics of African culture as the 'communal nature of existence of African families' which to a high degree assists the sick at home however this culture may also prohibit the sick-person from advanced planning as it is considered going 'against the culture'. This may put pressures on professional care providers who are limited in their interventions in respect of the families' wishes. It is equally true that access to state-of-the art hospitals in Africa may not always be the case and thus there may not really be a choice for carers to opt-out of the role. In fact Zaman et al. (2017) explain that in Sub Sahara Africa most palliative care is provided at home by informal carers mostly women but this may include elderly and children. Kumar (2013) describes similar situations in India, where the access of patients to qualified medical care is very low and even lower services are available for palliative patients. Although where services exist these are considered as excellent. However with the work of civil society, patient groups and the community services have improved in Kerala. Speaking of India one cannot but remember the work which is carried out by the Missionaries of Charity, the religious order founded by St Teresa of Calcutta in 1950. Although it is not a patient organisation, in the absence of family or any carers, the order cares for impoverished ill and aging people in more than 130 countries. The Kalighat, the Home of the Pure Heart formerly known as the Mother Teresa's Kalighat Home for the Dying Destitutes is a free hospice for the poor. Although this place is criticized as not offering the best healthcare in the World, the Missionaries of Charity, still claim that the give the poor the opportunity to die with dignity in according with rituals of their faith, some people would have lived a life of animals but at least receive a humane death.

Various Palliative organisations and Hospices have specific mechanisms to help carers during the time they are caring for terminally-ill patients. These may offer respite or relief services so that carers can take time-off for themselves in-order to look after themselves. As the Victoria Hospice states '*it can be difficult to care for another when you don't care for yourself'.* Hospices in Western Countries and Australia offer training programmes and online support for carers. Chapman (2013) explains how professional nursing or palliative care services can support carers care for their terminally ill at home. Learning from other conditions is important, an interesting training programme made available by the WHO for carers is the WHO iSupport program (Alzheimer's Disease International, 2018). This is an online training program targeted for carers of people with dementia. iSupport was developed by WHO in collaboration with academics but also with valuable contribution and advice by Alzheimer's Disease International and other patient organisations, experts, people with dementia, and carers. Dementia can be diagnosed at early stages however being a progressive disease one is bound to face end-of-life care issues. This training programmerecognised the fact that caring for a person with dementia, be it a family or a friend can be demanding, stressful and tiring thus the programme targets to teach carers to take good care of themselves. The training covers 5 main areas (1) What is dementia; (2) Being a caregiver; (3) Caring for me; (4) Providing everyday care, and; (5) Dealing with challenging behaviour. www.iSupportForDementia.org

Expertise Each patient is first and foremost an individual person, and as the term implies, every person has an inherent unique perspective on life, especially what he/she considers meaningful and equates as his/her life. Patients, who seek to engage in patient organisations, will arguably nearly always do so for one reason only, because they think that more work needs to be done at an institutional level to improve the lives and better the experiences of those patients who will come after them. This aspect of patient advocacy is very interesting since it highlights the altruistic rationale behind patient activism. While medical professionals will do their best to provide therapeutic and physiological support, it would be quite a simplistic view to uphold that illness only affects the biological aspect of the individual. Those affected by a condition will have a unique perspective which can never be fully understood due to its uniqueness. Patients will live with the condition continuously, acquiring skills and self-management tips and tricks along the way, which although sometimes might seem unorthodox from a scientific perspective, they will suggest and share enthusiastically amongst fellow sufferers. Autonomy effectively implies that every person is tasked with being self-directive, and most of the time, medical professionals can only contribute in a limited manner to those factors which will ultimately influence decisions. Patients' organisations are crucial in order to provide an accessible platform where networking and sharing of expertise between patients can take place in a safe, non-judgmental environment. When patients do not have access to such network groups, this affects negatively the overall experience (Civan et al. 2009), therefore ensuring that patients' organisations are supported and well organized should be a top priority when looking at policy recommendations and infrastructure. The need for institutions to recognize the invaluable input that can be provided directly by patients needs to be a factor when it comes to health care professional-client relationship and representation, especially in the areas of policy development. Using patient recorded outcomes and feedbacks as tools that guide policy development is extremely important so as to ensure that the patients' voice is not only heard but listened to.

Within the Expertise argument it is very relevant to consider the contribution of the non-professional carers helping the patient during this time. There is a very interesting balance which would need to be reached between the patient and carers, who decides about what, where and how much. The patient and the carers should be very active participants in the caring team together with professionals who are caring for the patient within their specialty however it is a challenge to work together for the patient holistically and not in bits and pieces. Fendler et al. (2015) base their very interesting argument on team practices in relation to terminally ill cardiac patients where services may not always be very equipped for such conditions. They argue about the fact that palliative care does not mean 'giving up' or 'accepting death' but rather how support can be given to patients where their condition is beyond any available treatment, is chronic and life-limiting.

An interesting model called 'integrated multidisciplinary model' for care is presented by Fendler et al. (2015) where the patient and non-professional carers (caregivers) are central to the care plan and these are supported with 'layers' of professionals and support givers according to need. The professional aspect is composed of relevant specialties according to the stage of the illness and others may be included as need be. But the professionals' role is key in supporting the patient as best as can be. Apart from medical guidance such situations may require decisions of planning death at home vs end-of-life care in a hospital setting.

Engagement is defined by EPF (2015a, b) as *patients need to be involved in designing more effective healthcare for all, and in research to deliver new and better treatments and services.* The role of patients' organisations in helping patients and their carers throughout their illness is very diverse but patients' organisations are very active in providing education opportunities and resources for patients. Patients' organisations based at local and national levels are assisted by technology, with various programmes, web-based training seminars and podcasts made available to people irrespective of their condition and health situation. The most important thing is literacy especially digital literacy and access to an electronic device. Whilst the voice of individual patients is important and they can be powerful advocates based on their own personal experiences and circumstances, when patients come together in patient organisations their voice becomes stronger. Patients' organisations can act as representatives on a policy level and in a much broader perspective. The WHO (2015) includes shared decision making through active involvement of patients in taking decisions about their health, in considering options including the choice of taking no action, in pondering risks and benefits and in analysing how the available options suit the patients' values and preferences. The indication of choices may be made in an informal manner through advanced planning or in a more formal legal way through advanced directives. It is important to note that the strength of documented patients' wishes may be based on the mental capacity of the patient. This matter may not always be a clear cut position between medics and lawyers thus in taking decisions one needs to ensure that the patient is given the full information and is competent enough to express ones' own decision.

One cannot approach the topic of Patient Empowerment and the active involvement of patient groups without dealing with advanced directives. These are a set of instructions completed ahead of time for your family and/or care providers to use if you are ill or injured and unable to speak or make decisions about the medical treatment you want to receive. Advanced Directives are sometimes also known as a 'living will'. Soto-Perez-de-Celis et al. (2017) stress the point that Advanced directives are legal documents which express the patient's decisions about end-of-life care and are drawn up when the patient has full mental capacity to express their wishes about treatments and interventions should the need arise in the future when they are incapacitated or unable to make decisions themselves. The importance of having a robust policy which effectively addresses the advanced directives cannot be highlighted enough. Advanced directives need to be discussed in terms of autonomous choices. Disregarding the fact that 'second order' autonomy issues will always affect choices (Frankfurt 1987; Beauchamp and Childress 2001), it is important that policies are designed in a way to enhance autonomy of service-users. The main function of Advanced Directives is to allow the patient to be able to decide in advance his/her preferences as regards treatment, whilst he/she is still competent to express his/her wishes (Capron 2009). It is important to remark at this point that although from a legal perspective, advanced directives are usually framed as negative rights (right to refuse treatment, rather than a right to choose a type of treatment), from a humane point of view, Advanced Directives should also take into consideration the patients' preferences as regards the type of treatments available at various stages. Having a well-structured policy does not only enhance the autonomy of the patient but it also safeguards all parties involved, since having something to guide the professionals in charge of the end-care stage removes the burden from having to either decide according to the practitioner's interpretation of best interest, but also avoids unnecessary burden on the patient's relatives. As with all autonomous choices, for an Advanced Directive to be valid there needs to be a clear line of communication between the patient and professional. Although there is always a risk to circumstances varying from when they are discussed to when they actually occur, giving the ability to the patient to clearly express himself/herself on what he/she considers acceptable or not, helps everyone involved to provide a personalised approach to care.

Although historically Advanced Directives have been around since 1967 (Nanovic 1990) there is yet no established universal standards guiding such a process. Advanced Directives have been include in US Federal legislation in 1991 whilst the Council of Europe included the concept of Advanced Directives in 1997 in the Convention of Human Rights and Biomedicine (Soto-Perez-de-Celis et al. 2017). Patients' organisations come in all shapes and sizes but two core objectives nearly always stand out, patient education and provision of support regardless of geographical location. Resources and literature available to assist organisations in education campaigns are quite scarce, and from a practical perspective, the differences in approaches to Advanced Directives are so huge that collaboration between international organisations in education campaigns is not feasible. The absence of a universal agreement on a rigid framework has been shown to be a major source of frustration to everyone involved, and it is one of the main barriers to a more expansive implementation (Lovell and Yates 2014). The issue of assisted dying has further complicated the discourse around Advanced Directives, since it increases the divide between countries when it comes to end-of-life care. The importance of having adequate patient representation whenever policies regarding Advanced Directives are discussed, ensures that the rights of all the parties involved are safeguarded.

An important aspect which is sometimes not given enough attention when Advanced Directives are discussed is the issue of providing psychological assistance throughout the whole journey. Psychological support and counselling, does not only help with managing stress but it also helps patients to better articulate their emotional adjustment to the experience. Counselling will also address the psychosocial aspects of the illness, and facilitate communication with the family and relatives. Disenfranchised and ambiguous grief present in such situations where loss is experienced before someone effectively passes on, might also impact Advanced Directives where it is more loosely structured and relies more on power of attorney representation (Lund et al. 2015). Advance planning will not only include therapeutic options but also more personal preferential options which are not strictly clinical in nature. There also exists another dimension to advanced care directives, which concerns a better utilization of resources by avoiding excessive interventions which may be considered excessive by the patient himself. This aspect is a sensitive aspect and from an ethical perspective care must be taken not to descend into comparing values which are incommensurable.

Equality Equality is defined (EPF 2015a, b) as *the need for patients to be supported to become equal partners with professionals in the management of their condition.* As already mentioned, when navigating through the complexities of factors affecting patient experiences, cultural barriers, and consequently, resistance to remove these barriers, play a very important part. Emanuel and Emanuel (1992) identified four main possible relationships, which range from the paternalistic, collaborative, interpretative and deliberative model. From a patient's perspective achieving equality between professionals and patients is the minimum prerequisite for having a meaningful rapport rather than a transaction between two opposing parties. Navigating through options by discussing them in a meaningful way, rather than bombarding the patient with raw data is indeed a bit more lengthy and laborious, but it is arguably the right approach from a moral perspective. Equality is a key factor in patient empowerment since it effectively recognizes that the relationship is not that of the expert versus the lay person, but rather a friendship model as described by Aristotle (1999) in his Nicomachean ethics (book eight) where reciprocity would ensure that in order for the relationship to be virtuous, this 'friendship' is not based on utility or pleasure, in other words not motivated by any prospect of material gains. When approaching equality between parties in an end-of-life scenario, although undeniably all the medical staff involved will have total commitment and dedication towards those who are under their care, the Freudian notion that we rationalize death while unconsciously clinging to immortality (Freud 1957), may be a mechanism whereby medical professionals cope with the enormous task they have of being responsible for the wellbeing of the patient during the last leg of their journey. Therapeutic boundaries are useful from a psychological perspective, but failure to realize that these boundaries have been blurred usually affects negatively the patients involved. Self-awareness of professionals involved is important, because being able to realize when emotional over investment is occurring, noticing changes in attitudes and language directed towards patients, or having the urge to control choices of patients is a sign that the relationship might be harmful to the patient. In circumstances where there may be issues of conflict between professional and patient Patients' organisations will not be hindered by this boundary and they can effective contribute to the equality balance. Soto-Perez-de-Celis et al. (2017) whilst outlining various models which exist in Latin America conclude their argument with a statement which is valid globally; the discrepancies which exist in service provision and legislation about end-of-life between different countries and even within pockets of society within the same countries leads to inequalities. Thus in times when resources are limited a societal approach to timely investment in primary and secondary prevention should be taken up together with education to potentially reduce the burden of mortality rates.

Attempts to drive policy have been sprouting in this millennium. The WHO has been issuing several documents and recommendations to have adequate palliative and end-of-life policies in place by governments for various years. This is mostly applicable for developing countries but not only as the concept of dying is universal (WHO 2015). The article quotes Dr. Belinda Loring, from WHO's department for Management of Noncommunicable Diseases, Disability, Violence and Injury Prevention, *"Palliative care must be available to all people, of all ages, with all diseases,"*. Kumar (2013) outlines an excellent example in Kerala, India, where despite the difficulties like in other regions, the initial work by the local community, volunteers and civil society, they drove to have a Palliative Policy developed which includes specialized training for doctors and professionals coupled with voluntary support within the local patient groups and local community to ensure safe supply of food, water and medicines to the terminally-ill.

There exists quite a divide when it comes to the current models utilized across the globe. Similar to other areas in medicine, some countries are more developed than others when it comes to frameworks and models. A positive framework which has been moving on a European level is the SIP Platform (Societal Impact of Pain Platform) (https://www.sip-platform.eu/en) which started in 2009 to bring to the attention of the European Commissioner, member states and civil society to get together to reduce the societal impact of pain in the EU. Over these years SIP has hosted various symposia involving all stakeholders and produced policy papers promoting a bottom-up approach to get administrations and politicians to tune-in to the needs of citizens and act. Surely the issue of Chronic pain is very close to end-of-life issues since it is certainly an experience of many when all attempts at a cure have been exhausted often people have to endure the burden of pain on a daily basis. The reality of assisted dying becoming increasingly available has also further muddled the role of palliative health care, since arguably there is the gradual attrition and replacement of the tenet 'to do no harm' with 'first and foremost relieve suffering'. This makes it easier to dismiss the often more complex palliative care path, and not provide the necessary infrastructure to address the issue of pain and suffering by arguing that euthanasia is providing the solution. The roadmap proposed by SIP(Malta) (SIP 2017, pg 42) highlights the proactive role such patient organisations have in this regard. Their approach to address the subject in an objective manner, undertaking scientific research in collaboration with experts and reliable data collection to back their arguments, essentially ensured that the proposals were factual. The resulting roadmap essentially lays the foundation and groundwork for governments and policy makers to address this issue, thus facilitating the process whilst also providing the possibility to access a network of relevant stakeholders in the consultation process from the very beginning.

Whenever official policies are lacking or are not effective, the power of patient organisations emerges to meet the needs as these examples highlighted by WHO (2014). Casa Sperantei is a Romanian example of an institution which was founded as a charity in 1992 and was crucial in changing the cultural perceptions associated with palliative care and directly affecting policy development by establishing minimum standards for palliative care services. Another example of patients driving change in the palliative care model is that by Hope Hospice, a community based palliative care model which provides service to those that for some reason are not eligible for sponsored care in the United States. They pioneered the concept of access for all and various patient-centred initiatives like bereavement counselling and care, delivered through a multidisciplinary team approach. Hope has implemented an array of coordinated care programmes, each with its own staff, that focus on quality of life through palliative care. In Tanzania the community is the responsible agency that offers the *Continuum of care for persons living with HIV/Aids* (CHAT), which provides education as well as direct palliative care support to sufferers.

13.3 Conclusion

Different countries will have different approached to end-of-life care. Patients' organisations and communities have historically contributed by providing a haven to patients while things got formally organized at an institutional level. Hospices are an embodiment of the philosophy that seeks to provide a 'holistic comforting' by utilising a palliative approach towards the end-of-life stage. From a systematic analysis perspective, there is so much fragmenting and compartmentalization that makes it difficult to generalize (Jimenez et al. 2018). Patients' organisations have long recognised that when it comes to end-of-life care, sustainability of services is one of the most crucial aspects that will affect successful outcome. Sustainability is dependent on two core factors: education of patients so that they are knowledgeable in their rights, and sufficient provision of health care professionals, which are adequately trained in their specialized field. The responsibility of national health systems to respond in a timely manner with adequate provision and resources as early as possible linking it to prevention, early detection and treatment programmes is highlighted by WHO (2018). The action should span between professionals and society at large and thus patients' organisations have a core mission in achieving these goals.

The services provided by patients' organisations go far beyond than just providing a service to the patients themselves. Patients' organisations are uniquely placed to offer realistic and practical recommendations based on actual experiences of those they represent. Patients' organisations are vital when it comes to highlight unmet needs and unsatisfactory service. The scope of patients' organisations essentially entails that the patient is at the centre of every recommendation, thereby implying that such recommendations are not dependents on constraints usually affecting institutions. Involving patients' organisations also increases transparency during policy drafting and reduces inadvertent paternalism when it comes to policy. The interdisciplinary team approach to end-of-life issue, should ensure that all aspects of preference based options are explored by the patient. Recognising that the clinical aspect is but a small, albeit a very crucial, part of the factors influencing the end-of-life journey is an important step. Tapping into such a resource should be a priority for every institution, as well as for individual clinicians. Differing models of healthcare and health services should not mean that there is also a differing value associated with preferences patients. Clear communication is key, but it should be followed by implementation to facilitate the expressed wishes of the patient.

References

Alexander Morgan Capron. 2009. Advance directives. In *A companion to bioethics*, ed. Ed Helga Kuhse and Peter Singer, 2nd ed., 299–311. West Sussex: Wiley, at p300.

Alzheimer's Disease International. 2018. *From plan to impact*. London: Alzheimer's Disease International (ADI).

Aristotle. 1999. Friendship between unequals. In *Nicomachean ethics*, ed. T. Irwin, Book Eight, viii: 1159a9–60a9, 127–129. Indianapolis/Cambridge: Hackett Publishing Company.

Astrow, A.B., G. Kwok, R.K. Sharma, N. Fromer, and D.P. Sulmasy. 2018. Spiritual needs and perception of quality of care and satisfaction with care in hematology/medical oncology patients: A multicultural assessment. *Journal of Pain and Symptom Management* 55 (1): 56–64.

Bai, M., and M. Lazenby. 2015. A systematic review of associations between spiritual Well-being and quality of life at the scale and factor levels in studies among patients with cancer. *Journal of Palliative Medicine* 18 (3): 286–298.

Balboni, M.J., A. Sullivan, A.C. Enzinger, Z.D. EpsteinPeterson, Y.D. Tseng, C. Mitchell, et al. 2014. Original article: Nurse and physician barriers to spiritual care provision at the end-of-life. *Journal of Pain and Symptom Management*: 48400–48410.

Beauchamp, T.L., and J.F. Childress. 2001. *Principles of biomedical ethics*. Oxford: Oxford University Press.
Canadian Hospice Palliative Care Association. 2004. *Quebec End-of- Life Palliative Care Policy*. [ONLINE] Available at: http://www.chpca.net/media/7856/Quebec_policy.pdf. Last Accessed 23 Feb 2019. Available in French at: http://publications.msss.gouv.qc.ca/msss/fichiers/2004/04-828-02.pdf. Last Accessed 23 Mar 2019.
Chapman, S. 2013. *A good death at home: Home palliative care services keep people where they want to be*. [ONLINE] Available at: http://www.evidentlycochrane.net/a-good-death-at-home-home-palliative-care-services-keep-people-where-they-want-to-be/. Last Accessed 23 Feb 2019.
Civan, A., D.W. McDonald, K.T. Unruh, and W. Pratt. 2009, May. Locating patient expertise in everyday life. In *Proceedings of the ACM 2009 international conference on supporting group work*, 291–300. ACM.
Consistency,' Dick L Rev 95 (1990): 209–234, at pp. 211–212.
Emanuel, E.J., and L.L. Emanuel. 1992. Four models of the physician-patient relationship. *JAMA* 267 (16): 2221–2226.
European Patients Accademy for Therapeutic Innovation (EUPATI) [ONLINE] Available at: https://www.eupati.eu/. Accessed 27 Feb 2019.
European Patients Ambassador Programme (EPAP) [ONLINE] Available at: https://www.europeanlung.org/en/projects-and-research/projects/european-patient-ambassador-programme-(epap)/home. Accessed 27 Feb 2019.
European Patients Forum (EPF). 2015a. *EPF Background Brief: Patient Empowerment*. [ONLINE] Available at: http://www.eu-patient.eu/globalassets/campaign-patient-empowerment/epf_briefing_patientempowerment_2015.pdf. Accessed 23 Feb 2019.
———. 2015b. *Patient Empowerment Campaign*. [ONLINE] Available at: http://www.eu-patient.eu/campaign/PatientsprescribE/. Accessed 02 Feb 2019.
———. 2017. *Toolkit for Patient Organisations on Patient Empowerment*. [ONLINE] Available at: http://www.eu-patient.eu/globalassets/library/publications/patient-empowerment%2D%2D-toolkit.pdf. Accessed 23 Feb 2019.
Fendler, T.J., K.M. Swetz, and A.A. Allen. 2015 July. Team-based palliative and end-of-life Care for Heart Failure. *Heart Failure Clinics* 11 (3): 479–498.
Frankfurt, H. 1987. Freedom of the will and the concept of a person. In *The importance of what we care about*. Cambridge: Cambridge University Press.
Freud, S. 1957. Thoughts for the times on war and death. [(II) Our attitudes towards death.] Strachey J, Freud A (trans.). *The Standard Edition of the Complete Psychological Works of Sigmund Freud*, 289–300.
Gire, J. (2014). How *death imitates life: Cultural influences on conceptions of death and dying*.
Gysels, M., C. Pell, L. Straus, and R. Pool. 2011. End-of-life care in sub-Saharan Africa: A systematic review of the qualitative literature. *BioMed Central Palliative Care* 10 (6): 1472–684X.
Ilemona Ekore, R., and B. Lanre-Abass. 2016. Aftican cultural concept of death and the idea of advance care directives. *Indian Journal of Palliative Care* [Online] 22 (4): 369–372. Available at: https://www.ncbi.nlm.nih.gov/pmc/articles/PMC5072226/?report=printable Accessed 6 Jan 2019.
Jimenez, G., W.S. Tan, A.K. Virk, C.K. Low, J. Car, and A.H.Y. Ho. 2018. Overview of systematic reviews of advance care planning: Summary of evidence and global lessons. *Journal of Pain and Symptom Management*.
Kuhse and Peter Singer. 2009. 2nd Ed, 299–311. West Sussex: John Wiley & Sons.
Kumar, S. 2013. Models of delivering palliative and end-of-life care in India. *Current Opinion in Supportive and Palliative Care* 7: 216–222.
Lovell, A., and P. Yates. 2014. Advance care planning in palliative care: A systematic literature review of the contextual factors influencing its uptake 2008–2012. *Palliative Medicine* 28 (8): 1026–1035.

Lu, Y., Y. Gu, and W. Lu. 2018. Hospice and palliative care in China: Development and challenges. *Asia Pac J OncolNurs* 5: 26–32.

Lund, S., A. Richardson, and C. May. 2015. Barriers to advance care planning at the end-of-life: An explanatory systematic review of implementation studies. *PLoS One* 10 (2): e0116629.

Mallia, P., Laferla, G., Aquilina, K., Agius, E. (2017) Consensus statement on end-of-life ethico/legal issues. [ONLINE] Available at:https://www.um.edu.mt/__data/assets/pdf_file/0010/322768/pdfCONSENSUSSTATEMENT_20JUL1714.pdf. Accessed 14 Jan 2019.

Nanovic, S.J. 1990. The living will: Preservation of the right-to-die demands clarity and consistency. *Dickinson Law Review* 95: 209.

Online Readings in Psychology and Culture, 6(2). https://doi.org/10.9707/2307-0919.1120.

Phelps, A.C., K.E. Lauderdale, S. Alcorn, J. Dillinger, M.T. Balboni, M. Van Wert, T.J. VanderWeele, and T.A. Balboni. 2012. Addressing spirituality within the care of patients at the end-of-life: Perspectives of patients with advanced cancer, oncologists, and oncology nurses. *Journal of Clinical Oncology* 30 (20): 2538.

SIP. 2017. *Proceedings Structured Cooperation between Health Care Systems tackling the societal impact of pain! #SIP2017*. https://www.sip-platform.eu/files/editor/events/SIP/2017/Proceedings/SIP_Proceedings_2017v1.0_with%20links.pdf. Accessed 14 Jan 2019.

Soto-Perez-de-Celis, E., Chavarri-Guerra, Y., Pastrana, T., Ruiz-Mendoza, R., , Bukowski, A. & Goss, P.E. (2017), End-of-life Care in Latin America J Glob Oncol. 2017 Jun; 3(3), 261–270.

Victoria Hospice. *Preparing for Death – A Guide for Caregivers*. [ONLINE] Available at: https://www.victoriahospice.org/i-am-caregiver/preparing-death-guide-caregivers. Accessed 14 Jan 2019.

Winkelman, W.D., K. Lauderdale, M.J. Balboni, A.C. Phelps, J.R. Peteet, S.D. Block, L.A. Kachnic, T.J. VanderWeele, and T.A. Balboni. 2011. The relationship of spiritual concerns to the quality of life of advanced cancer patients: Preliminary findings. *Journal of Palliative Medicine* 14 (9): 1022–1028.

World Health Organisation. 2009. *WHO guidelines on Hand Hygiene in Health Care*. [ONLINE] Available at: https://www.ncbi.nlm.nih.gov/books/NBK144013/pdf/Bookshelf_NBK144013.pdf. Last Accessed 23 Feb 2019.

———. 2014. *Global Atlas of Palliative Care at the End-of-life*. Worldwide Palliative Care Alliance. [ONLINE] Available at: https://www.who.int/nmh/Global_Atlas_of_Palliative_Care.pdf. Last Accessed 23 Feb 2019.

———. 2015. *Palliative care: for all ages and all diseases*. [ONLINE] Available at: https://www.who.int/features/2015/south-africa-palliative-care/en/. Last Accessed 14 Feb 2019.

———. 2018. *Palliative care leaflet WHO*. [ONLINE] Available at: https://www.who.int/en/news-room/fact-sheets/detail/palliative-care. Last Accessed 14 Feb 2019.

World Health Organisation, Europe. 2015. *Engaging patients, carers and communities for the provision of coordinated/integrated health services: Strategies and tools* [ONLINE] Available at: http://www.euro.who.int/__data/assets/pdf_file/0004/290443/Engaging-patients-carers-communities-provision-coordinated-integrated-health-services.pdf?ua=1. Last Accessed 14 Feb 2019.

Zaman, S., H. Inbadas, A. Whitelaw, and D. Clark. 2017. Common or multiple futures for end-of-life care around the world? Ideas from the 'waiting room of history'. *Social Science & Medicine* 172: 72–79.

Chapter 14
Developing Pathways Towards Improving End of Life Care and Advanced Planning

Pierre Mallia

Abstract Hospitals, institutions and even whole countries have different problems when dealing with end of life care. In the west there may be lack of access to formal palliative care; in poorer countries there may be more concern about lack of basic medications such as morphine, or even worse, lack of water and proper sanitation. The chapter addresses how to bring teams together to develop ongoing pathways to improving end of life care by identifying issues, discussing frustrations, and developing a plan of action to tackle particular issues.

Keywords Hopsitals · End-of-life care · Pathways · Identifying problems · Organising · Review

14.1 Introduction

Hospitals, institutions and even whole countries have different problems when dealing with end of life care. In the west there may be lack of access to formal palliative care; in poorer countries there may be more concern about lack of basic medications such as morphine, or even worse, lack of water and proper sanitation. The latter are public health issues which the World Health Organisation agonises on. This is intended as a model which can be used by institutions and hospitals up to (or involving) governmental bodies. The chapter addresses medical leadership intending doctors, and other health care professionals to involve themselves in processes they detect and which indeed may cause frustration. Medical leadership calls for people to go beyond their normal call of duty and involve themselves in action which improves outcomes for patients. Besides giving more meaning to individuals, rather than a sense of frustration, it also makes sense professionally to improve systems. Professionalism involves doctors as healers, patient-partners, and team workers,

P. Mallia (✉)
Medical School, University of Malta, Msida, Malta
e-mail: pierre.mallia@um.edu.mt

P. Mallia et al. (eds.), *Challenges to the Global Issue of End of Life Care*,
Advancing Global Bioethics 17, https://doi.org/10.1007/978-3-030-86386-9_14

and together with other HCPs as managers and leaders, patient advocates, educators and innovators (Tweedie et al. 2018): "Innovations may be in technology, health systems, health policies, health financing, how health care is delivered, how doctors' work is organised, and much else".

The main objective in this chapter is to show how leadership can effectively be used to organise groups which meet in retreats (or summer schools), rather than short seminars, in order to get health care professionals together to discuss the needs of their hospital or area and formulate a plan towards achieving these goals. The example taken is *Advanced Care Planning at the End of* life. The retreat in turn forms a curriculum (Mallia 2015–2018). intended to address the necessary skills which may be needed. It is acknowledged that more developed countries may differ considerably in their needs. The model used in the Erasmus+ EndCare project is used (Ibid.).

Therefore, whilst the global intention of the chapter may be used to address issues which are more to do with public health – such as clean water – the example being presented addresses the needs of professionals working in hospitals or institutions and bringing thoughts together to develop a curriculum of training and to formulate paths which address those needs in which high authorities are needed. Studies in the EndCare project done at Mater Dei Hospital, Malta, showed, for example, that many health care professionals, including doctors, appreciated training in palliative care, and where absent, wished they were given this specific training (Abela and Mallia 2016a, b, c). The summer school encouraged group work which pointed to the need of good communication skills, a knowledge of the law, a knowledge of moral issues, including respective religious beliefs, better training in palliative care etc. It also pointed to the necessity of formulating plans (pathways) to assess whether existing legislation covers accepted moral principles, such as being able to remove extraordinary treatment, or, giving more pain relief, without the fear of litigation. Doctors showed more concern with litigation whilst nurses showed more concern for knowledge of moral issues, and patient education in this regard. This resulted in meeting with the Minster for Health, who happened to be a Paediatric surgeon, who took a great interest and moved towards working to create a Hospital Ethics Committee and better end of life care. Indeed, it is a demonstration of the ripple effect where the Bioethics Research Programme recognised the need for better end of life care and took it upon its programme to apply for the Erasmus+ project which in turn can a great impact. The process is ongoing.

Towards this end the chapter is divided into two sections, each or all of which can form part of the retreat. The first section addresses pathways towards implementation of the needs addressed in these retreats/summer schools and addresses the curriculum design. The report is reproduced with the permission of the coordination team. The second section discusses useful systems approaches and quality assurance for implementation.

14.2 Case Presentation: *Developing Pathways for End of Life*

One of the eight outcomes of the EndCare project was *A Pathway to implement change at political level for advanced care planning, especially in countries where such planning does not exist.* One of the partner countries, Malta, was used to develop and test the model.

The stages involved:

1. Studies to show the need
2. Applying for funds – Erasmus
3. Summer schools
    (a) To define the problem
    (b) To look as cases
    (c) To identify a needs assessment
        (i) Knowledge of law
        (ii) Knowledge of moral theory
        (iii) Knowledge of different religious values
        (iv) Communication skills
        (v) Conflict resolution
        (vi) Proper palliative care practice
        (vii) Need for a Hospital Ethics Committee
    (d) To create a curriculum for training
4. To formulate a pathway
    (i) Further research
    (ii) Further retreats or summer school
        1. Reports
    (iii) Implementation at political and administrative level
        1. Hospital Ethics Committee
        2. Meeting with Minister for Health
        3. Dissemination of project
        4. Meetings with hospitals
        5. Consensus Document (Faculties)
        6. Media
5. Planning further summer schools
6. Implementation
7. Quality assurance

14.3 Historical Context

The EndCare project originated through experiences of Health Care Professionals in Malta who had concerns about the lack of harmonisation within Mater Dei Hospital (the national hospital) on how end of life is managed. Palliative Care is not consistent and specialists do not necessarily have special training in the area. Moreover the Palliative Care Unit is seen as a unit where patients are transferred for the last days and continue to be seen by the consultant of the patient, although there is a resident consultant in the ward.

On the other hand, some time before the application for this project, the crises with the Liverpool Care Pathway (LCP) had developed. Annex 3 contains The definitions of the LCP and the pathway developed to arrange the situation in a document entitled *One Chance to get it Right*. The title of the document can be seen as a misnomer in the sense that the country only had this one chance. This was not the case. In effect the title means that *with each patient we only have one chance (to get it right)*. Once the patient dies that chance is lost.

The LCP was a palliative care pathway for people in whose area no hospice was available. The latter are charities and therefore exist mostly in middle and upper class areas and tended to be less frequent in the lower socio-economic areas. The government implanted this scheme with good intentions of providing adequate end of life care. The pathway also had training implemented in it. However the media caught on complaints about its implementation and although it was accepted as part of the NICE guidelines for end of life care, it came under attack. Some people felt that their relatives were simply put off all treatment including hydration and nutrition and that this amounted to euthanasia. One consultant even spoke out against it.

At the time the Bioethics Research Programme of the Medical School of the University of Malta invited the chairman of the Ethics Committee of the Royal College of Physicians (RCP), Professor John Saunders, to speak in defence of the pathway. Of course he acknowledged that the difficulty was in lack of its understanding and lack of training by specialists. But it *was* a pathway, in the sense that it was not a tick-box of what should be done. Guidelines were written on when and how treatments were to be stopped. It was a path. The lesson learnt from the LCP experience were several:

1. Good intentions alone are not enough
2. Neither is developing a pathway
3. Training of physicians and nurses was essential
4. Education of patients, family and public on how the pathway works is important.
5. 'Marketing' is therefore an essential tool which health care often tends to omit.

The *One chance to get it* right report, commissioned by the National Health Service of the UK (NHS), involved also a patient grow and together they formed the Leadership Alliance for the Care of Dying People. Little is known to this day what has really changed within the pathway itself. Rather it was an exercise of involving people beyond health care and seeing that it was implemented well. The pathway itself was therefore theoretically sound. Its implementation was in general good as well in a vast amount of hospitals and many patients died comfortably. But the cases, which also seemed frequent, where the pathway was not implemented well, caused the public concern and later outcry.

The pathway described here takes into consideration that it is not enough to implement a route to change and change itself. It must be diffused in its educational potential to professionals and the public and it must be audited and reviewed periodically. This is shown in the schemes which will follow.

The following are some example of concerns observed or expressed:

- A nurse on call called the junior doctor in the evening to give pain relief to a dying patient who was in distress and was known to be dying. The doctor, not having any instructions on the notes, hesitated and did not increase the dose of morphine as it will cause respiratory suppression and hasten the death of the patient.
- A consultant neurologist who was treating a dying patient with 'mad-cow disease', noticed that the patient was continuously removing his oxygen mask. Since the patient was recognised to be dying he discussed with the relative, who in turn accepted, that he would be removing the mask as the patient seemed uncomfortable. A nephew however got to know – he was also a doctor and working in Germany – and reported that this was tantamount to euthanasia. The magistrate on call later reported that the doctor did nothing wrong after not only considering the law but after consulting an ethicist. The neurologist however relinquished the patient to another consultant who then acceded to the changed concerns of the family and who put on the mask again.
- Whilst on a radio programme the lead of this project, a doctor and ethicist, heard a patient complain that 'her mother was killed because of that last dose of morphine she was given'. She stated that her mother had died about 15 min later.

The above cases each show a different problem in end of life care. The first shows a lack of training not only of individual doctors but also in how communication between professionals when the death of a patient is imminent is not implemented. The second shows how lack of communication skills and proper management of end of life, including lack of understanding on what is and what is not euthanasia both on the part of health care professionals (HCPs) and the public lead to misunderstandings. It also shows that consultants can have their decisions challenged and one ought to question why one has to resort to transfer a patient to another doctor. The third case shows lack public education about end of life care.

One should reflect a little about the second and third case. Malta is largely a Catholic country and even non-practicing Catholics will usually be aware of the values they were brought up in. Clearly the Catholic Catechism states that pain relief can be given as part of ordinary care even if it hastens death. Conversely if a treatment is seen either as futile or in any way causing discomfort, is disproportionate, or in any way deemed by the patient to be seen as extraordinary, then it need not be given. Clearly the Church authorities had to be included in any project contemplating end of life care, not only for its input, but also to be encouraged to teach and educate the public about what is allowed. Removing futile or extraordinary care is not passive euthanasia for the Catholic Church, as some are prone to describe it.

Around the same time a patient with Motor Neuron Disease (ALS) did not wish to spend his life in an undignified way when he was to be completely dependent on his relatives or others. He therefore petitioned the government to introduce legislation in favour of Euthanasia. A public debate ensued and contemporarily a Parliamentary Social Affairs Committee discussed the issue inviting the public, patient groups and experts. More interestingly however were the so-called Vox-Pops done on television programmes discussing the issue. Many people said 'no' to euthanasia and many other (more than expected), said 'ye'. But when the patter were asked why most did not refer to rights but said statements like, 'Why should one die in pain', or, 'why should one not be able to refuse treatment'.

14.4 Towards the EndCare Pathway

Clearly there was lack of education on the part of the public. In fact the patient with ALS was subsequently shown that he had a right to refuse even life-prolonging treatment, such as being put on a respirator, and allowed to die a natural death comfortably – meaning in effect that he could be sedated so that he does not die in distress. After all this is what is done to patient dying from lung cancer or severe obstructive airway disease who enter hospital with respiratory distress in their final hours. Although relatives seem to see that patients have improved because they do not see the former signs of distress, in reality the patient is simply being kept comfortable and the distress treated. This lack of communication also causes some concerns.

To this effect and Erasmus project was contemplated by the Bioethics Research Programme to study this issue. The objectives were to use the Summer School as a learning ground not only for the professionals or public attending but also for the project team as well in order to be able to create a tool which can be used in institutions or countries to better conditions offend of life. Studies done in the beginning of the project showed that there is lack of a clear and harmonised understanding of end of life care, more especially palliative care, amongst HCPs. Even more so was the lack of education amongst the public. But the former studies also showed that whilst nurses were more concerned about the lack of public (and their own) understanding of the moral principles underpinning end of life, doctors on the other hand were more concerned about medico-legal issues and the lack of clarity in the law about whether they can legitimately remove futile treatment and/or give pain relief.

This set the scene for what was to be studied:

1. Summer schools to include
    (a) Sessions discussing cases on end of life care and concerns of the individual participating.
    (b) Discussing pathways to how these can be managed
    (c) Talks on communication skills, spirituality, the law, palliative care, what is futile and extraordinary care etc. These were to serve for people to reflect on what may be lacking.

2. The development of a curriculum, through the learning experience of the summer school, of a Pathway – which was to be a plan of action to study issues, implement change and review periodically.
3. Implement any changes to the law
4. Issue a Consensus Document between the faculties of Medicine & Surgery, Laws, and Theology.
5. Encourage, through the same pathway, Advanced Care Planning (ACP).

These were goals for the local scenario but were to serve as a tool for the publications of the project and its dissemination. They were to be incorporated within the eight outcomes of the project.

14.5 Defining Steps

The Pathway was divided into three main steps.

14.5.1 Step 1 – Identifying the Problem

This step identifies the problem. A problem with end of life can be realised through personal experience or any other venue. The important thing is that one notices that the issue was not an isolated one. A recurring problem, such as lack of giving adequate pain relief to dying people, or, fear of removing futile treatment because of lack of awareness either by HCPs or public are thought of.

At this stage one can discuss problem with colleagues or at other venues to identify and raise further awareness. It is important that the problem is felt by many. Professionals follow easier if they somehow have met with or thought about the problem themselves. This can be done during events, courses, union meetings, staff meetings etc.

It is important to be opportunistic. A media event or an event such as the request for euthanasia by a patient triggered considerable discussion. Questions usually followed – why is it that people believe they are dying in pain or that they have no right to refuse treatment. Is this true? Is there a lack of public education? Is there are lack of consistency in treating people approaching the end of their lives?

At this stage, collecting evidence is important. It is useful going to administration, ministries, etc. without actual evidence that the problem is an issue. Politicians especially may be moved by the media (and opportunism in this regard can be useful). But failure of this necessitates the collection of evidence. This can be done by questionnaires and should be done professionally and if possible published. The published article will also give impetus to the problem, even if in medical journals. It may not be wise however to involve media lest one antagonises those from whom one needs to ask. Rather the media ought to be allowed to catch on.

Collecting of evidence pushes people from simply talking about an issue to doing something. Ideally one identifies a small team of people to plan ahead. Research can be done with the aid of people doing a dissertation for a Masters degree, through projects etc. Before one can do this the second step is necessary however.

14.5.2 Step 2 – Organising the Retreat

It is important to collect colleagues and organise, through funding, CPD or otherwise a discussion of the problem. If the problem is diffuse people will attend. It is here that the 'fire' is lighted – people (are allowed to) vent out the problem. It is important in these events that a facilitator (not the chairperson) is there to collect ideas on flip chart or something similar. This shows people that their ideas are being acknowledged and noted. A summary is made.

The retreat ought to be a series of meetings. This can be done in a summer school or on periodic events. During these events the people continue to discuss the solutions. *The Curriculum* can be useful here. People ad HCPs learn more about the problem of end of life: the law, the social issues, patient groups, what religious and other social institutions say, communication skills, medical leadership etc.

The problem can now be broken down into needs, e.g.:

1. The need for a communication skills course
2. The need for further research and how this can be done
3. The need to involve medication
4. The need for clarity in legislation
5. The need that the Church teaches what can and cannot be done at the end of life rather than speak out against euthanasia only. i.e. education about what is *not* euthanasia
6. Etc.

14.5.3 Step 3: Organising a Path (Way)

Here a strategy is drawn up. It is important that one identifies the coordinators and the members of the group, if there is any. However it is easier if there is a distribution of labour. Ideally team work will not allow someone to be identified as the protagonist which may lead some people to feel they will not be acknowledged. Although this should not be the case as we are dealing with a real issue and is about patients, everyone is all too human and not acknowledging human needs according to Maslow's hierarchy can lead to loss of good individuals. Also when potential audiences from administration to politicians listen to 'we' rather than 'I', it has more motive force.

The pathway itself brings what the Retreats in Step 2 have identified. In the case of the end of life harmonisation pathways done in Malta it was the following:

1. Defining clear Aims and Objectives (which breaks down the general Aim into parts), and Collection of evidence
2. A consensus document between the faculties of medicine & Surgery, Laws and Theology on end of life. (Theology was involved due to the cultural nature of the issue).
3. Funding – e.g. further structural funds after this Erasmus project finishes. It was recognised that involving groups outside hospital was important and this set the preparation for EndCare 2 in the future to follow on.
4. Presentation to
   (a) Minister for health
   (b) President of the republic
   (c) Archbishop
5. Seminars and conferences to raise further awareness and disseminate.
6. Publishing of articles etc.
7. Defining outcomes (Figs. 14.1 and 14.2)

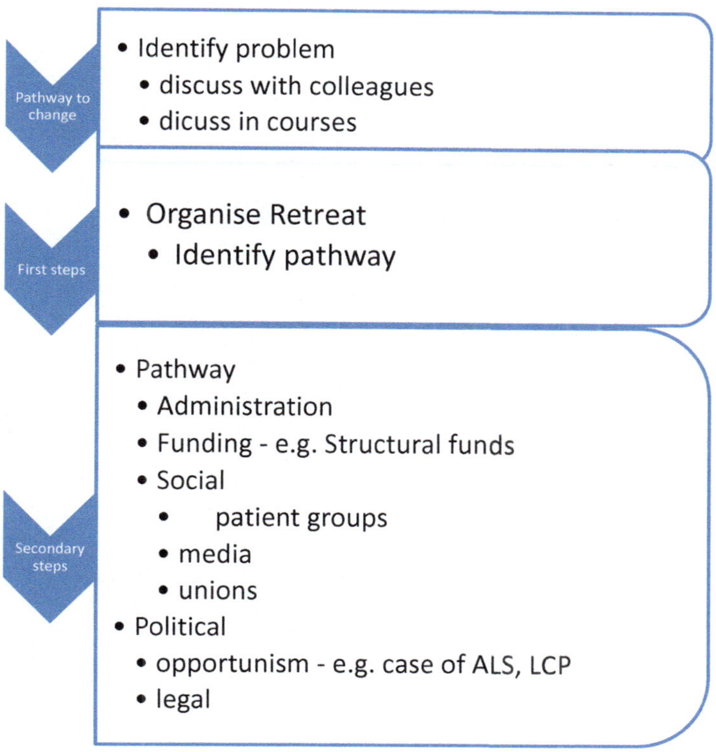

Fig. 14.1 General Scheme for preparing for a Pathway to resolve End-of-Life issues

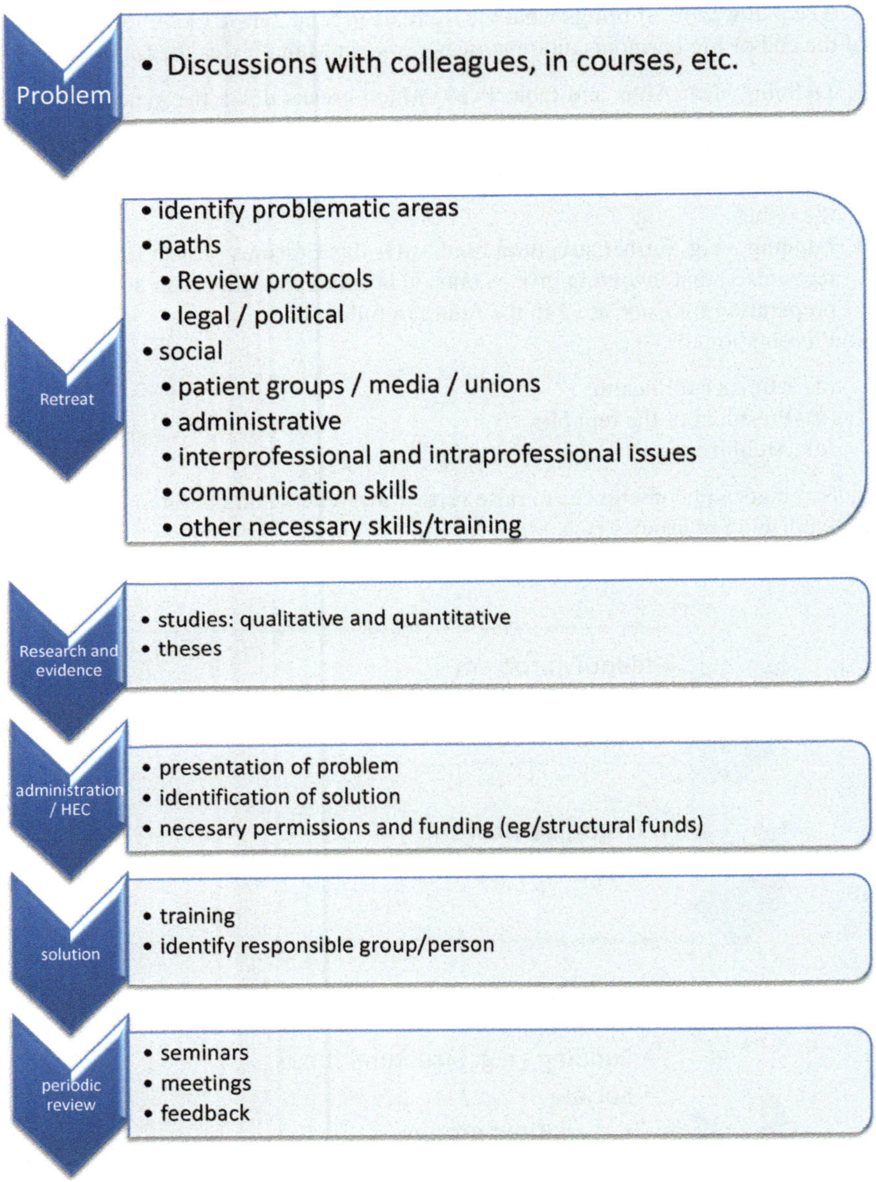

Fig. 14.2 Elaborate scheme on the three steps

14.6 Periodic Review Proposal

Figure 14.3 shows how the process does not stop and one needs to come back to the original problem periodically and seeing whether objectives are being achieved and if not why. It is important that after a year (or month), for example, people feel that we have moved on the problem. What has been done? Have the goals for this year ben achieved? If not, why?

One has to stop and re-evaluate. This review process examines the conscience of the group. A member who motivates may be important. Are we thinking beyond our personal work and home life? Are we being medical leaders in our field? Are we finding *meaning* in our profession by being protagonists in effecting change?

Often enough people attend meetings to do with union issues because they want better conditions for work. Unions can be involved if necessary but one has to be careful if one wants to politicise the issue or not, which may have its advantages and disadvantages – whilst one may be biting the hand that feeds him, one may also be making space for political predators to use your experience as a weapon. This may

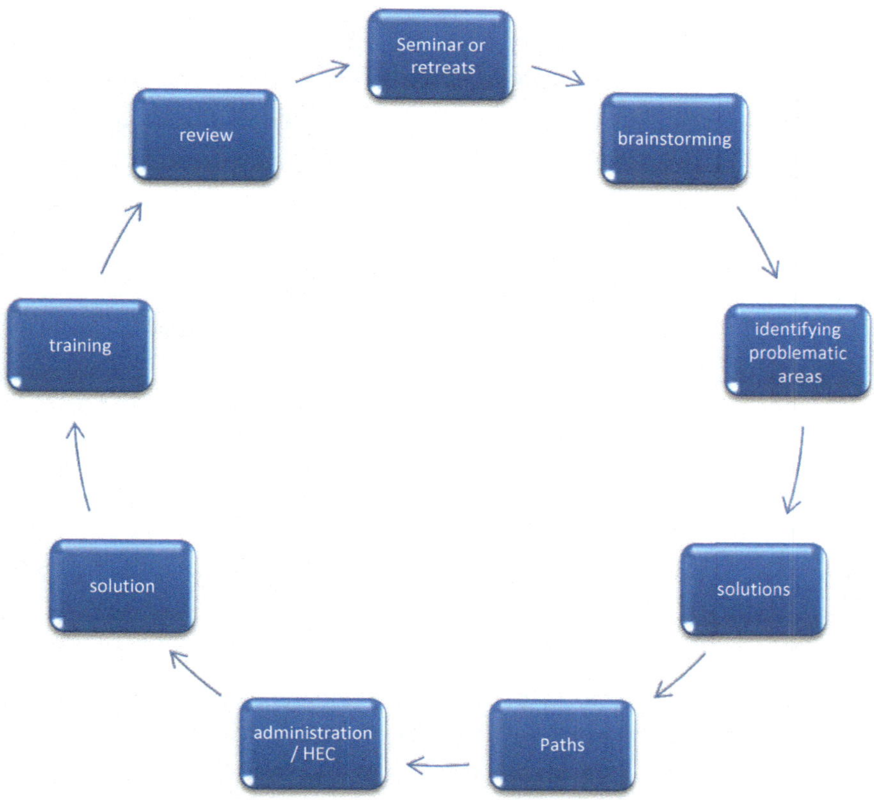

Fig. 14.3 Pathway review cycle

compromise the project. The project should be in equipoise and seen to be honest and trustworthy. It is a place where the virtue ethics of the profession must come out. It also has to be the place to unite HCPs. If the issue is politicised, some may leave because their party is being condemned and others may join as long as their party is gaining.

Finding meaning in one's work also by working beyond one's ward gives leadership and responsibility to people. They stop being helpless and simply thinking that 'they' (whoever they is) should solve the problem. Medical leadership means being involved.

14.7 Results

In the case of Malta, the following results were achieved and effected the beginning of change from Ministry level to down to the main hospital. The list includes:

1. A Series of published papers and manuscripts.
2. A consensus document which was disseminated throughout hospital
3. Meeting with the hospital CEO
4. Meeting and presentation to the Minister
   (a) Minister in turn took interest and promised to bring to attention of parliamentary group to see which laws were needed
5. Collaboration between faculties of laws, Medicine, and Theology to clarify moral, legal and medical aspects through above document and through Seminars and Conferences
6. Invitation of international speakers to share their experience
7. Pathways for a curriculum for future workshops/conferences (SEE APPENDIX)
8. Summer school of the project
   (a) This generated further interest. Some People who attended also came to the summer school of L'Aquila and Dublin
   (b) Consultants who attended requested that these school be repeated in their own departments. In particular future retreats or summers schools were requested by:
      (i) Department of Anaesthesia
      (ii) ITU
      (iii) Dept. of Oncology
      (iv) Hospice movement
      (v) Members of the Malta Health network also showed interest. This network was found to have an enthusiastic new chairperson.
   (a) Courses and lectures on end of life were introduced in existing Masters Course
   (b) Masters and Law students were encouraged to do their dissertations on end of life in order to further study the issue. These were collected.

(c) A meeting with the Archbishop was held by the Coordinator which was very useful in creating awareness that people should be though what can be useful at the end of life according to the teaching of the Church. Reassurance that the project was not introducing euthanasia but introducing right to refuse treatment deemed extraordinary by the patient, and proper end of life management including pain relief and furthering palliative care was emphasised.
(d) Whether due to the project pathway or not, it was useful that the Church, following the promise to build a Hospice for palliative care after the debate on euthanasia, actually moved and gave a building to the Hospice movement.
(e) The Hospice movement in turn sent for the coordinator of the project to introduce training and a Masters degree under his aegis at the medical school.
(f) Preparation for EndCare2 which will be extended to the community: family doctors, patient groups, social institutions, education etc. to improve condition for dying at home.

14.8 Systems Approach

Formulating a pathway can involve not only change in medical practice but a revision of systems. Indeed, the topic of Systems can be a module in a curriculum design for a particular place of country. The Royal College of Physicians has recently looked at how systems can help change (Dean 2019a). The editor notes that systems of care are very local and context specific and that what works for one place may not fit or work for another, even within the same country (Dean 2019b). Whilst the editorial acknowledges that data and evidence-based design are important as portrayed here, the concepts of deigning curricula is only indirectly referred to in other articles within the publication and discussed within the context of training. Of course, all training needs two thing – some form of curriculum design, and a selection of what topics are important to learn, apart from the design of the system itself. Thus, a different style of communication skill may be necessary for training people in group consultations than when dealing with patients individually (Jones et al. 2019). The RCP has built a Quality Improvement group (RCPQI) which aims to make quality improvement more accessible (REF Dean). It can easily be seen how these aids aimed for the UK can help also on a global level (Figs. 14.4 and 14.5).

On a different level the concept of supply and demand is recognised with health economies (Kanagaratnam et al. 2019). However, 'complex health and social needs, associated with an aging population, pose a novel challenge to NHS resources and in particular, its workforce'. We recognise here the parallel countries sense on a global level with regard to end of life. The Workforce Repository and Planning Tool (WRaPT) process is a novel patient centred approach to workforce planning (Ibid.). The authors claim that the tool enables a new type of workforce modelling with the assumption that 'changes to the workforce are predicated on changes in activity'. The steps (Fig. 14.6) aims to address key challenges facing the UK. It is a good tool to address the supply for the demand in improved end of life care. The process

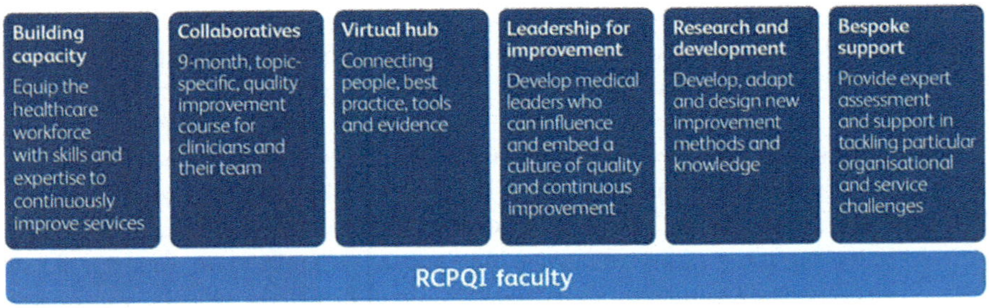

Fig. 14.4 Royal College of Physicians Quality Improvement programme workstreams. (Dean 2019b)

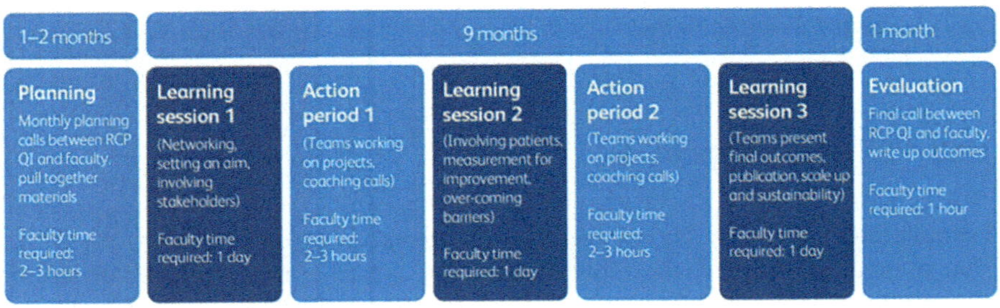

Fig. 14.5 Structure for collaboratives to deliver training. (Dean 2019b)

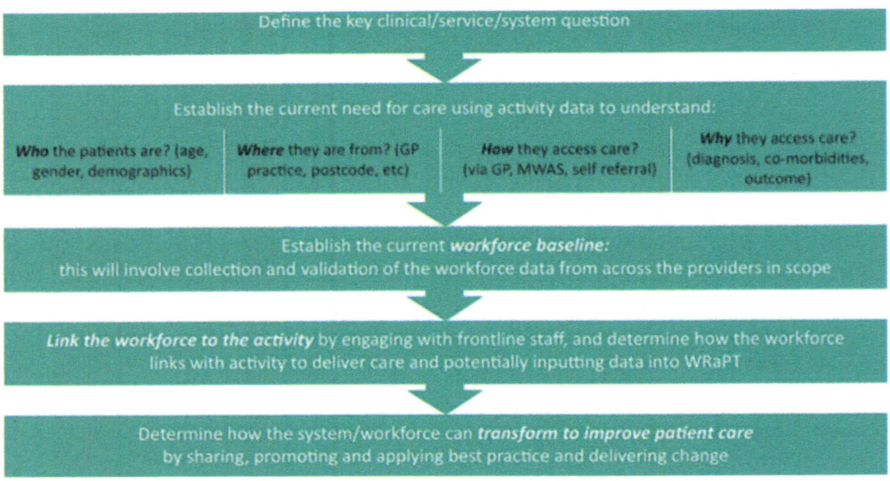

Fig. 14.6 The Workforce Repository and Planning Tool (WRaPT) process for workforce transformation. *GP* general practioner, *WMAS* West Midlands Ambulance Service, *WRaPT* Workforce Repository and Planning Tool. (Kanagaratnam et al. 2019)

involves five stages starting with discussions with organisation leaders and health practitioners (analogous to the Retreat method proposed in EndCare) to define the key questions. It then combines clinical observation and workforce data analysis using software tools identifying areas of *activity-workforce mismatch* giving evidence-based opportunity for movement of the work force to appropriate areas. The authors state that the primary difference between this model and other methods of workforce planning is the adoption of emerging tools to data evaluation, known as the realist view (Ibid.).

14.9 Quality Framework

If one does not learn lessons from other countries, one is bound to repeat them. The Liverpool Care Pathway (Chap. 3) provides a good lesson of how developing guidelines is not enough (Saunders 2013). One needs to oversee implementation and assure its quality. It can often be the case that one considers one's work done by producing a document or guidelines. This is not the case and medical leadership involves continuing to take responsibility throughout the process. Otherwise one simply finds oneself with a document which remains just that. People need to be trained to implement the document, others need to study feedback from HCPs and patients, etc. Assuring quality is the mechanism used in health care which makes the difference between a successful project and one that is bound to fail. It keeps the original members of the retreats involved if they so wish and the best reassurance of quality is to see the implementation of the process and work. The British responded with the document *One Chance to Get it Right*(Leadership Alliance for the Care of Dying People 2014). Indeed, with a dying person there *is* only one chance to get it right with them – which is what the title really means. One looks forward to future studies to assess the impact of that report. Yet Britain is a highly organised country and leads by example. There is no fear to criticise pathways, as with the LCP. In other countries obstacles may be political, transparent, cultural etc. Each country must form the pathway and curriculum which addresses *their* needs. But without an ongoing process to oversee that what was decided upon gets implemented and without a continuous assessment of the outcomes, one may easily fail. This is the purpose of the quality framework.

Countries ought to strive to have quality frameworks for proper end-of-life care and palliative care. Implementing pathways with due training and communication, for example, can give rise to distorted perceptions, as happened with the Liverpool Care Pathways. In point of fact, the lack of training and not following the 'path' may have made these perceptions right in some instances, as many British authors pointed out retrospectively.

As discussed in Chap. 9 Quality frameworks are important to link scholarship with action. Quality Improvement (QI) is a priority in health care. New research redefines best practice and health needs in particular populations, in this case those in whom death has been recognised as imminent. Moreover, it was pointed out that health needs in different countries change and this points towards important QI programme which needs to be adapted locally.

It was noted that there are other stake holders in end-of-life care, including nurses, other health care professionals, patient groups, legislators, hospice movements etc. and last but not least the politicians who are entrusted with effecting change. Broad consultation is needed to improve quality of care; also, Quality means that one has to focus on competence at all levels, from that of individual health professionals, to working as a team pointing towards the need of clear and concise templates or pathways, training in these pathways, clear defining of the roles within the team, with regular face-to-face meetings and regular professional development.

14.10 Conclusion

Frearson points to the importance of Hospice training and discusses how first year foundation doctors in the study felt that their medical practice was affected significantly when placed in Hospices pointing towards the usefulness of increased importance of placement of young doctors (in this case) in Hospices (Frearson 2019). Globally this can be adapted according to what means are available in countries – homes for elderly, hospices, palliative care, community medicine for those dying at home, etc. Frearson's qualitative study showed that at this level doctors can, Learn about Communication, Prescribing at the end of life, How to take a palliative history, Recognising death, Management of complex palliative patients, Understanding of hospices (or other settings) and palliative care as a specialty, The value of a good death, How to write discharge summaries, and Procedures used in palliative care and end of life situations. Within the context of EndCare Abela and Mallia showed that Vocational Training Programmes for doctors (in this case the community) appreciated considerably the module and placements of Palliative end of life care (Mallia and Abela 2011).

The time spent in creating pathways at the end of life is well spent. One ought also to consider end of life care in specific disaster/pandemic situations such as the recent COVID pandemic where many dying people, especially elderly were dying alone. Such situations are difficult but with the post-mortems of such situations, one can prepare for these eventualities for those unfortunate enough to die a slow death in such circumstances. Of course, without having systems of end of life care in place in more normal circumstances, one cannot then delve into the more mundane or strained situations. Pathways have been deemed useful to create more economically viable systems such as the group consultations mentioned in this chapter, albeit respecting patient outcome. But pathways are not only utilitarian models. They ought to be also deontological. The EndCare project was conceived because it was deemed untenable that different consultants approach end of life in different ways and that there was no harmonised system to treat patient equally and as humanely as possible. The evidence collected in the preliminary phases of preparing for pathways also points out to discrepancies which are discovered incidentally – such as bad communication on files and record between doctor-to-doctor, and nurse-to-nurse, for those on 24-h duty who see patients of other firms. Clear pathways also point to what concerns different professions more, from legal to ethical and moral issues, communication skills and systems. Every journey starts with a first small step. Perseverance even of one person will build a team and recognise the needs of particular settings and countries. But ideas do not have legs and pathways do not fall out of the sky. Ideas change along the way until a harmonised approach can be devised and implemented.

References

Abela, J., and P. Mallia. 2016a. Maltese Doctors' views and experiences on end of life decisions and care. *Maltese Medical Journal* 28 (2): 16–26.

———. 2016b. Maltese doctors: Views and experiences on end of life decisions and care. *Maltese Medical Journal* 28 (2): 16–26.

———. 2016c. Training in palliative care medicine and maltese doctors: A cross-sectional survey. *Journal of the Malta College of Family Doctors* 5 (2): 13–19.

Dean, J. 2019a. Evidence-based care systems design – part 2. *Future Healthcare Journal, Royal College of Physicians* 6 (1): 3–4.

———. 2019b. Update from RCP quality improvement: quality improvement faculty and partners network. *Future Healthcare Journal, Royal College of Physicians* 6 (1): 6–7.

Frearson, S. 2019. Perceived educational impact, challenges and opportunities placements for foundation year doctors: A qualitative study. *Future Healthcare Journal, Royal College of Physicians* 6 (1): 56–60.

Jones, T., A. Darzi, G. Egger, J. Ickovics, E. Noffsinger, K. Ramdas, J. Stevens, M. Surnego, and F. Birrell. 2019. A systems approach to embedding group consultations in the NHS. *Future Healthcare Journal, Royal College of Physicians* 6 (1): 8–20.

Kanagaratnam, S., S. Dholakia, J. Wood, A. Monkhouse, D. Wood, K. Abelak, and J.P. Jeans. 2019. The WRaPT process – a novel and patient-centred approach to workforce planning by a clinically active workforce. *Future Healthcare Journal, Royal College of Physicians* 6 (1): 21–24.

Leadership Alliance for the Care of Dying People. 2014. *One chance to get it right*. London: Gateway Publications.

Mallia, P. 2015–2018. *EndCare. On harmonisation and dissemination of good practice at the end-of-life*. Project no. 2015-1-MT01-KA203-003728.

Mallia, P., and J. Abela. 2011. An evaluation of the palliative care module in the specialist training programme in family medicine. *Malta Medical Journal* 22 (4): 26–33.

Saunders, J. 2013. The Liverpool care pathway. *Journal of the Malta College of Family Doctors* 2 (2): 5–10.

Tweedie, J., J. Horden, and J. Dacre. 2018. *Advancing medical professionalism*. London: Royal College of Physicians.

Chapter 15
Conclusions

Pierre Mallia, Nathan Emmerich, Bert Gordijn, and Francesca Pistoia

Given the advances made in the biomedical sciences across the twentieth century and that continue today one could assume that we are in possession of a proper definition of certain fundamental concepts, such as life and death. However, if anything, these same advances have contributed to a great deal of uncertainty surrounding death and how we ought to understand it. Can a person in a chronic vegetative state be the object of therapeutic obstinacy, when the chances for recovery are extremely poor? Are those born with severe anencephaly sufficiently alive to be declared dead? Are those we assess as brain dead already dead or do they die once we cease providing life support or perhaps a short time afterwards? The law requires that medical doctors record a time of death not least because, as Lamb puts it '[i]t is as wrong to treat the living as dead as it is to treat the dead as alive.'[1]

[1] D. Lamb, 'What is death?' in R. Gillon (ed.) Principles of Health Care Ethics. Chichester, UK: John Wiley and Sons, 1994.

P. Mallia (✉)
Medical School, University of Malta, Msida, Malta
e-mail: pierre.mallia@um.edu.mt

N. Emmerich
Australian National University, Canberra, Australia
e-mail: Nathan.Emmerich@anu.edu.au

B. Gordijn
Institute of Ethics, Dublin City University, Dublin, Ireland
e-mail: bert.gordijn@dcu.ie

F. Pistoia
Neurological Institute, University of L'Aquila, Coppito, L'Aquila, Italy
e-mail: eliana.close@qut.edu.au

P. Mallia et al. (eds.), *Challenges to the Global Issue of End of Life Care*,
Advancing Global Bioethics 17, https://doi.org/10.1007/978-3-030-86386-9_15

The implication or, perhaps, operative presupposition is that there is a bright line between life and death. However, even if this is the case, it is far from clear that we or medical science can identify specific criteria that will allow us to determine when it has occurred. Clearly, the reign of the cardio-pulmonary standard is long over. With the onset of CPR and life-support systems we have confused this basic phenomenological notion of death which all seems to understand. We can resuscitate someone, which literally means 'bring back to life', and continue to perform cardio-pulmonary physiology beyond a certain established time. There is of course a reason why an established time of 15 min is stipulated. Beyond that there is too much damage to the brain for life to be considered. Yet if we go beyond, and this is the case for many countries, some patients live but albeit most in a persistent vegetative state. There is very little chance for someone to come out of this state but the very fact that some do makes many hold on to the possibility and tell doctors not to switch off their loved ones' machines.

Not only can we resuscitate patients and thereby restart hearts that have stopped beating we can, at least in some circumstances, remove a patient's heart and replace it with another. Equally, whilst the notion of brain death might be uniquely modern,[2] in the sense of representing an alignment between science, medicine and culture, it is not without its problems.[3] Which definition should we embrace: whole, stem or neocortex?[4] Perhaps we should just accept death as a 'wickedly complex' problem, something that can only be properly understood when illuminated from a number of perspectives and, therefore, cannot be reduced to a singular definition.[5]

As troubling as the definition of death has proved to be, it would be a mistake to think that resolving it would solve the kind of issues that arise in medical practice and health care at the end of life, (especially on a global scale where the issues may not simply be about prolonging life or disproportionate treatment, but not having even morphine, or, for that matter, basic necessities). Pace the above cited quotation from Lamb, we should recall that not only is it wrong to treat those with a prospect of recovery as if they could not be helped, it is just as wrong to treat those who cannot be helped as if they had a prospect of recovery. Thus, being able to recognize when death is imminent and unavoidable would be of more use than any definition, no matter how philosophically and scientifically robust it might be. Perhaps of even more use would be a broader cultural disposition to *accept* death when it is unavoidable or when nothing more can be done to improve the patient's condition. We might then be able to focus on how to take care of dying patients. Whilst people may expect more in hospital, we need to remember we are treating a person and causing

---

[2] Vidal, Fernando. 2009. 'Brainhood, Anthropological Figure of Modernity'. *History of the Human Sciences* 22 (1): 5–36.

[3] Truog, R. D. 2007. 'Brain Death-Too Flawed to Endure, Too Ingrained to Abandon'. *The Journal of Law, Medicine & Ethics* 35 (2): 273–281.

[4] Zaner, Richard M. 2012. *Death: Beyond Whole-Brain Criteria*. Springer Science & Business Media.

[5] Emmerich, N. 2016. 'The Deaths of Human Beings'. *QJM: An International Journal of Medicine* 109 (4): 229–30. https://doi.org/10.1093/qjmed/hcv195

discomfort for the simple reason of making the family think that we are doing everything to 'keep the person comfortable', or for some other reason, is certainly unethical, no matter how much we try to justify it. But certainly we would have to consider whether the discomfort of poking a person with a needle is really necessary. After all it may take several attempts to find a non-collapsed vein, and even a subcutaneous drip may cause the discomfort of the swelling of the tissues being filled with fluid and not being drained as quickly.

Trying to keep people alive as much as possible, not only through CPR, but also by attempting extraordinary, disproportionate, and even futile treatment, has distorted, to say the least, our acceptance that death is imminent or present. Death has indeed become the enemy. This is an accepted course of action for doctors when people are involved in accidents or unexpected injuries. We try our best not simply to fight death but to help the person through such time as to allow the body to recover. This was the original purpose of life support systems. Thus, in the case of Karen Ann Quinlan, the doctors kept the girls on life support in the beginning in the hope of a recovery. But since the brain-death criteria had been developed, when it was evident that her brain had suffered too much damage for her to recover the parents naturally questioned this behaviour. They were Catholic and saw the procedure as interfering with 'God's plan', as it were. They legitimately questioned, 'Then why are you keeping her on life support?'. One has only to imagine the un-sensical reaction to the answer, 'Because she is not yet brain dead'.

It is not, of course, that we are congenitally unable to recognize, accept or discuss death and dying. Indeed, caring for dying patients is a major component of the medical specialism, palliative care. What is required is a broader acceptance of the kind of medicine and care palliative care has to offer. Indeed, a broader acceptance of its particular perspective or underlying philosophy.[6] Whilst we tend be preoccupied with the possibility or simply the idea of a cure there is no reason why we cannot move past or modulate our hopes and expectations when it becomes appropriate to do so. We need not take extraordinary or disproportionate steps to preserve life at all costs when it becomes clear that death, inevitable as it always was, draws near.

We have avoided the topic of euthanasia, not only because it is beyond the scope of this book and of the project (EndCare) from which this book has originated, but also because many advocate euthanasia in order to avoid pain or becoming dependent. Moreover, the topic of euthanasia also relates to patients who find themselves in a state which they find unacceptable, such as tetraplegia or the prospect of imminent dementia. As such, the argument is not really about the end of life as addressed in these pages. Here the concern is for patient's suffering during a terminal illness and the process of dying. They need not feel pain, they may be sedated if necessary, they need not accept extraordinary treatment and they have a right to refuse even life-prolonging treatment. Thus, someone with Motor Neuron Disease fear the state of being kept alive on a ventilator without being able to move, then they may indeed

[6] Randall, Fiona, and R S Downie. 2006. *The Philosophy of Palliative Care: Critique and Reconstruction*. OUP Oxford.

refuse this treatment. It is in regards these kinds of patients that we have recommended the global introduction of Advanced Care Planning, rather than discussed the broader notion of Advance Directives.[7]

Many have come to believe that we should continue to hydrate dying patients through intravenous line, and, when these become impossible to insert, via subcutaneous drips. Indeed, considering the fact that dying people tend not drink, and are even less likely to eat, whilst people dying at home rarely have such interventions, we should consider our underlying purpose. Perhaps not giving fluids during the dying process would avoids the arduous and discomforting task of evacuating. We do not know. If, as may well be the case, we are putting in a subcutaneous drip in order to appease the family, or to meet their expectations, this must be balanced against the potential discomfort being caused. Poking a person with a needle may not really be necessary and it may take several attempts to find a non-collapsed vein. Even a subcutaneous drip may cause discomfort by swelling the tissues being filled with fluid and not being drained as quickly. Whilst people may expect more in hospital, we need to remember we are treating a person and causing discomfort for the simple reason of making the family think that we are doing everything to 'keep the person comfortable' is unethical, no matter we might try to justify it.

On a global scale end of life brings different issues – from countries which provide too much to countries which do not have the bare minimum, such as morphine. The scope of this text was not in moral instruction which ought to be accepted on a global level, but to address the specific and contextual issues and to serve as a helpful tool. Professionals ought to find meaning not only in their daily work, but also in being the people who perceive the problems and then go on to try and find solutions. Getting health care professions together may be difficult and certainly there are cultural protocols which only the people of the country may know. Nurses in the western world may find themselves questioning certain actions but feel unable to do anything about it. Summer schools and retreats serve to provide a safe environment on critical thinking and using creative skills to provide solutions or pathways to solutions. One may recognise skills which are lacking in oneself or in colleagues. The retreats may provide a means of developing curricula for topics which may be necessary, such as understanding of the law, understanding of different moral values for different cultures, the needs for communication skills courses, the need for palliative care courses even for consultants and senior nursing officers. Of course, the topics will vary on a global level as the context changes. Things may take time to change. But working towards a particular issue provides the health professional, be her a consultant or nurse or any other health care professional, with more meaning and scope in improving the quality of life of those one is caring for.

---

[7] Of course, gaps remain: can a tetraplegic refuse to be medically assisted in feeding? Might they refuse feeding and ask to be sedated until death? Given the role played by medicine in placing such patients in this position it is right that medicine leave them to a motionless life? These are not, however, questions we have sought to address, at least not directly.

Appendix: A Curriculum for the Harmonisation of End of Life Care Within Micro or Macro Systems

EndCare, ERASMUS+ Project

Pierre Mallia

A Curriculum for Improving End of Life Care: An EndCare Erasmus+ Outcome

Introduction

'Modern affluent society is particularly uncomfortable with the reality of death, a discomfort that makes it a difficult area for both health care staff and patients and their families. Some doctors and nurses feel anxious about engaging in a conversation about death and prefer to avoid it….At the same time, some patients and their families find it difficult to face the thought of imminent death and understandable want 'everything possible' to be done, reinforcing the pressure on staff to adopt aggressive treatment approaches, however minimal the possibility of 'cure".[1]

[1] Ballatt, J., Campling, P. *Intelligent Kindness. Reforming the culture of healthcare*. Royal College of Psychiatry Publication (UK), 2013.

P. Mallia et al. (eds.), *Challenges to the Global Issue of End of Life Care*, Advancing Global Bioethics 17, https://doi.org/10.1007/978-3-030-86386-9

It is only over the last two decades that the term "end of life care" has come to be used with increasing frequency.[2] This reflects a growing concern with end of life treatment and care both on behalf of patients but more especially by health care professionals who witness daily activities which they may wish changed. In fact recently there has been and increasing number of books being published relating experiences of health professionals[3] and in turn an increasing number of books and literature on how EoL can be improved. This over-pours into the serious media.[4]

Not that end of life care has not been discussed before in the bioethics world. But somehow the concerns were more about euthanasia and its counterpart – palliative care. This is proving not to be enough. Clinical Ethics tends to need to move from the world of bioethics, which can be purely philosophical reflection. Health Care Professionals (HCPs) are concerned with giving people a 'good death'. This was indeed the experience of the Liverpool Care Pathway – a pathway with the good intention of providing palliative care services to those who did not have a hospice facility available (These being charities and therefore tend to concentrate around areas where they be more supported). The experience was negative and led to an avalanche and a revolution of end of life care in the UK. We believe we can all learn from this invaluable experience. The British have not tried to hide the problems but rather tackled them well. Not that there may not be room for such an opportunity for international 'growth' and learn from these experiences.

What essentially went wrong with the LCP was simple. People who were not trained in Palliative Care were the ones who were using it, even though they were qualified physicians. In many places, putting one on the pathways meant simply a tick-box of removing treatments, hydration etc, rather than assessing what needed to be done. It became known as a euthanasia pathway and indeed when referring to the LCP one still finds people, including people in bioethics, who saw it as an indirect purposeful euthanasia pathway.

The offset was the introduction of new NICE guidelines and the far more important Advanced Care Planning. It is imperative here to note that although many use or understand this term as being interchangeable with Advance Directives, there are inherent and important differences. An Advance Directive is a legal document which has been criticised that it may bring about a situation in which the patient, if deemed incompetent, may not change their mind. Conversely and Advanced Care Plan is a malleable tool and decision can change along the way. The important point is that the patient has a capacity to understand and retain information and give some form of feedback. Although all is noted and perhaps even (for legal purposes) require signature, it is not as legally binding as a document which can be written

[2] Hayes,A., et al. *Pathways through care at the end of life. A guide to patient-centred care.* Jessica Kingsley Publishers, 2014.

[3] See Resources: Gawande, Nitik Zitter, and O'Mahony

[4] Se, for example, *The Economist*, "How life ends. Death is inevitable. A bad death is not." April-May 2017, pp. 45-48.

years before someone actually has a disease. An ACP usually starts early on in a disease process.

We live in a social context of 'death-denial'[5] and many continue to treat till the very end without contemplating that any sort of palliative care or a change in plan. XXX relates an experience when she first had a CPR: the senior registrar was leaning against the sink with folded arms keeping an eye on the time and assessing the two junior doctors giving CPR. It was a dying elderly man already in kidney failure who was not put on a do-not-resuscitate (DNR) order. Although she was dying CPR was given. She could feel, with every push, the cracking of fibs, which in the elderly become brittle. To play safe the registrar continued CPR for 30 min (which begs the questions *who are we treating, the patient or the relatives? Are we giving good care or simply want to be legally sound to avoid litigation?).* After that he stopped the process. This was a life-changing experience for young doctor Zutik Zitter.[6]

It is not the first time that this 'flogging of dead horses'[7] has been criticised in renown journals like the British Medical Journal. The Royal College of Psychiatrists, in their publication *Intelligent Kindness* (REF), which, although dealing with the UK NHS, ought to be read by anyone interested in improving the experience of patients, write that the 'fear of reprisal' can lead physicians to do endless tests just so that they and their families believe that 'everything possible has been done'. This is simply wrong. John Saunders is quoted as saying that, 'at best CPR is the gift of life… followed by years of productive and fulfilled being…At its worst, it offers a scenario of vomit, blood and urine, then a confused, brain=damaged twilight, breathlessness from a failing ventricle, pain from rib fractures…until expiring in the thrall of the full panoply of intensive care or forgotten in the on-going darkness of the persistent vegetative state'. He rightly points out that no humane doctor would consider this a good death. It is the image of '*death in the industrial age*'[8] which is an automaton.

Interestingly Gawande[9] points out that when insurance companies in the USA started to offer palliative care as an option to continuous aggressive care, many patients opted for this. And indeed costs for the insurance did go down.

But the philosophy and scope behind the EndCare project and this curriculum as one of its outcomes is indeed to deal with the anxieties and the helplessness that HCPs, not least doctors themselves, feel in front of a system which seems cannot change. Indeed the UK experience has shown that system can change but it unfortunately takes a negative experience which gives bad media which in turn mobilizes

[5] Op. Cit., Hayes, p.14

[6] Nutik Zitter, J., *Extreme Measures. Finding a better path to the end of life*. Avery, new York, 2017. p.5.

[7] Ebrahim, S., "Do not resuscitate decisions: flogging dead horses or a dignified death?", *British Medical Journal,* 2000; 320:1155-6.

[8] Op. Cit., *Intelligent Kindness*.

[9] See Resources

politicians. What we can do is to create a tool whereby HCPs come together (and it is not excluded that patient groups can be involved) to 'trash out' the frustrations and problems, but then to seek to understand the underlying agendas and to work together to formulate a pathway – such as making a plan which can be put through associations and unions, which have the political clout and experience to induce politicians to effect change. We need to speak each other's language – and politicians certainly understand things in light of political philosophy and agendas. This was the LCP experience. LCP can be used as a warning sign to where good intention can lead if the system is perceived not to be working ideally.

1. Introduction to the curriculum

The scope of the curriculum is to bring together health care professionals working in end of life care in order to define and identify problems which exists within their hospital, locality, region or country. It is not excluded therefore that HCPs may invite patient groups, local representatives, administration and politicians to a part of their discussion.

2. Educational philosophy

A curriculum has been defined as an evolving animal (McEvOY); it changes according to needs. Each system has its strengths and weaknesses, opportunities and threats and participants are encouraged, to do a SWOT analysis as part of the process less they converge only on what each feels to be a problem. The model used is a combination of the Membership of the Royal College of General Practitioners (UK) and the Summative Assessment and Vocational Training for Family Doctors in Malta.

3. Aims and Objectives of the curriculum

Rather than identifying the problems participants have to feel that they are there as medical leaders, aiming to effect changes. The ultimate aim is the improvement of end of life care, be it in hospital, hospice, homes, or residences. HCPs experience and can hermeneutically tell when something is wrong. They bring this to the group in a retreat or meeting to see how the patients' experience can be less burdensome. The ultimate objective is therefore to understand the reasons for the underlying problems (for example, why doctors persist in giving treatment) in a non-blaming and non-threatening environment, and to come out with a pathways as a plan to implementing change, in the full knowledge that this pathway will take time and may involve the involvement of other expert participants. The ancillary objectives are defined in the outcomes below.

4. Definition of outcomes

   a. To have a clear understanding of the international and local standards of end of life care and the expectations as required by evolving international literature and guidelines.
   b. To be able to identify the problem being discussed, distinguishing it from ramifications.

c. To understand the underlying nature and to seek the true cause of the problem moving away from speculation.
d. To formulate a strategy or pathway to resolve this problem. This may be in the form of identifying training needs such as specific skills or to set a protocol or standard of care.
e. To take the opportunity to understand, revise, or update oneself on legal, moral and cultural issues at the end of life, communication, conflict resolution (*see Curricular content*).

5. Rationale of Modules

a. The modules have a particular order but institutions may decide to use then in an order which they deem more convenient, and. Based on module 1, they may find the need to omit certain modules.
b. Module 1 is an assessment exercise for the institution/s. It is a training plan to allow health professionals to exress their concerns, evaluate them, and indeed define them in perspective to see whether any change is necessary. Following this they will use Module 7 to develop pathways.
c. Modules 2 through 6 are put before module 7 as they are the most common problems identified which lead to a lack of harmonisation at the end of life. Hence there may be a lack of understanding or consensus on the medical and ethical approach between professions (both intraprofessionally, e.g. physicians may not feel the importance for palliative care specialists or training or updates, and interprofessionally where doctors and nurses, for example may have different perspectives on the patient and therefore the management – even though ultimately it is usually the consultant physician who is responsible. Then, legal and social issues have been found to be relevant, either because of lack of laws, or because of a lack of a clear understanding on how that law may be applied. Social issues include religious institutions which may be lacking in providing people with the proper moral teaching of their respective religions. However a module on spirituality emphasises that spirituality is not only about religion and that existential questions are faced by everyone.
d. It is felt that once problems at the end of life are faced and the team, or other people in larger contextual circumstances, come together to discuss the issues at hand, it is worth going through the other modules as they may well find that the issues have a wider perspective and that there may be other problems to face.
e. Finally we decided to include the UNESCO Bioethics Core Curriculum at the end. This is in fact a core curriculum respecting the Articles in the convention for human rights and bioethics. It will be necessary if it is felt that HCPs have not had proper courses in ethics. In this case, although listed as the 8th module, it can be done at any stage or concurrently.

6. Organisation of the curricular content

   a. Modules:

      i. Assessing EoL Care

         1. Strengths, weakness, opportunities, threats.
         2. Research at the EoL

      ii. Legal issues
      iii. Medical/Ethical issues

         1. Coordination
         2. Delivery of high quality care
         3. Futility
         4. What is extraordinary care
         5. Advance Care Plans
         6. Pain relief

      iv. Social issue – home, care
      v. Spirituality
      vi. Communication and Conflict resolution
      vii. Thinking about Pathways

         1. administrative
         2. Medical
         3. Political
         4. Social

   b. Template for modules:

      1. Title

         a. Reference document
         b. Date

      2. Introduction

         a. Rationale
         b. Local health care priorities

      3. Learning Outcomes
      4. Teaching and learning resources

         a. Work based experience
         b. Other learning opportunities

            i. Retreats
            ii. Workshops
            iii. Seminars
            iv. CPD

5. Formative Assessment

   a. Reflective diary
   b. Case discussions

6. References
7. Reference document used as a model
8. Further reading
9. Internet resource(s):

Module 1

1. Title: **ASSESSING EOL CARE IN THE CONTEXTUAL CONTEXT**
2. Introduction

Often health care professionals may not be content with the practice of end of life in their settings, which can be either the hospital in which they work, or their region or indeed the country. Certainly each system has its strengths and its weaknesses and change presents both threats and opportunities. There is certainly a perception that end of life needs to be improved and that it is a neglected 'core business' in medicine[10] and that it is inadequate.[11] There is also an awareness that training the next generation of doctors in palliative care is a key to bettering the future of end of life care.[12]

End of life care however is becoming a general issue world-wide and a lot of material in this regard is being published (see further reading). The change in the concept of autonomy and individualism may make people believe that 'everything that can be done should be done'. Certainly in the USA litigation on futile treatment,[13] in which doctors believe that they should not give further treatment whilst relatives dispute these decisions, leads courts in general to support the patients.

The aim of the module is to help participants explore the issue underpinning end of life . This can be done by formal studies and questionnaires to health care professionals, patient and relatives to explore issues like satisfaction, problematic areas, and logistical issues. Certainly some issues are at national level and will have to be tackled more broadly. But health care professionals are leaders in the medical field and their studies and assessments can lead to change. Other material such as reports, document, and indeed media coverage and published articles can also be formally studied and researched to tease out conclusions.

Conversely good records of decision processes and conflicts discussed can be fundamental in making retrospective and prospective studies on what actually goes on at the end of life.

3. Learning Outcomes
   a. To learn how to assess the quality of end of life care in the contextual context of regional or local settings.
   b. To understand the attitude of the general public, patients and relatives toward end of life and their understanding of laws, personal religious beliefs and other social factors which affect their decision

[10] Editorial, "*End of Life Care: the neglected core business of medicine*", The Lancet, Vol. 379, No. 9822, pp. 1171-1172.

[11] Kirchheimer, S., *"End of Life Care Inadequate"*, WebMD, http://www.webmd.com/health-aging/news/20040106/end-of-life-care

[12] Frist, W.H. et al, "Training the Next Generation of Doctors in Palliative Care is the key to the new era of Value-Based Care", in *Academic Medicine. Journal of the Association of American medical Colleges*, Vol.90, No.3, pp268-271. 2015.

[13] Veatch, R, "So-called Futile Care: The Experience of the United States" , in Bagheri, A.(ed) *Medical Futility. A Cross-National Study* Imperial College Press, 2013

   c. To study whether there is coherence in attitudes towards end of life amongst health care professionals
   d. To assess what legal structures are in place to protect health professionals and whether there is awareness of legislation or whether more needs to be promoted in this regard
   e. To learn how to evaluate the strengths and weaknesses of the setting and what opportunities and threats are faced. This will include legal, social (including cultural), and ethical aspects, communication issues, coherence in the system, and what courses of action may be done.
   f. To understand the importance of medical leadership in improving care.

4. Teaching and learning resources

   a. Retreats for interprofessional health professionals
   b. Group work
   c. Case studies
   d. Reading material
   e. Developing continuing professional development paths.

5. Formative assessment

   a. Reflective Diary
   b. Assignment on assessment of the setting discussed, either individual or as a group, describing the assessment process and the recommendations.

6. References

   a. End Care (Erasmus +) Protocol.

7. Further Reading

   a. Heath Iona *Matters of life and death: Key writings*, Radcliff Publishing, 2008.
   b. Gawande, A., *Being Mortal. Medicine and what matters in the end.* 2017
   c. O'Mahoney, S., *The Way we Die Now*, Head of Zeus Ltd., UK, 2016
   d. Nutik Zitter, J., *Extreme Measures. Finding a better path to the end of life.* Avery Press, New York, 2017.

8. Internet resources

   a. Palliative and End of Life Care Competency Tool: http://aiihpc.org/wp-content/uploads/2015/02/Palliative-End-of-Life-Care-Competency-Assessment-Tool-Sept12.pdf
   b. National Palliative Care Research Centre. Measurement and evaluation tools: http://www.npcrc.org/content/25/Measurement-and-Evaluation-Tools.aspx
   c. Evaluation and quality assessment of end of life care: https://www.caresearch.com.au/caresearch/ClinicalPractice/Physical/EndofLifeCare/EvaluationandQualityAssessment/tabid/742/Default.aspx
   d. Instruments. End of life Care Research Programme: http://depts.washington.edu/eolcare/products/instruments/

Module 2

1. Title: **LEGAL ISSUES**
2. Introduction

Legal issues at the end of life are often the concern of health care professionals.[14] In the United States courts have often awarded relatives of patients the right to futile treatment.[15] This practice has perhaps promoted the administration of extraordinary care and futile treatment to avoid conflict. However this continues to be bad practice. When it comes to CPR it has been dubbed as 'Flogging dead horses'.[16]

It is clear that health professionals may not feel that the law protects them and/or is favourable to good medical practice. Trust in the medical and nursing profession may also be at stake either way – over-treating or under-treating. This modules aims to help participants assess what their concerns are; whether they have a clear idea about the law; what guidelines exist in their respective communities and whether they find difficulty in communicating to patients and relatives about ethico-legal issues.

The module continues to help participant explore what needs to be done by formulating a concern to learn and disseminate guidelines and law; taking advice and formulating protocols, if necessary. Advanced Care Planning should be tackled as early as possible to allow time for understanding and reflection and to explain that it is all about having a good death. Conversely doctors ought not to continue with a so-called 'cure', creating false hope and not being able to discuss the imminence of death. There is perhaps the myth that 'doing all that we could do' is a good thing. Perhaps it avoids litigation or undue conflict but dying should be about the patient and not fear of conflict or the law.

Health Care Professionals should have a clear understanding of the law and, if absent, should seek that proper protocols are in place and guidelines for Advanced Care Planning for medical councils and hospital administrations. Participants are prompted to ask: do we have proper procedures implemented? Do we have ethics committees? Do I know whom to contact for help? Do I know enough about end of life palliative care?

3. Learning Outcomes

   a. Knowledge about the legal position on end of life in one's respective setting.
   b. Knowledge of what the respective medical councils and hospital administration say about approach end of life.
   c. Learn how to ask whether one is over- or under-treating a patient approaching death.

---

[14] Abela, J., Mallia, P.

[15] Veatch

[16] Flogging dead horses

d. Learn about the experience of the Liverpool Care Pathway and appreciate what can go wrong without discussing with patients and relatives and how a pathway or protocol should not be simply a 'to do' list but is a malleable tool and implemented according to need.
e. The legal dimension of proper standard of care about palliative care and the graphs that describe such an approach.

4. Teaching and learning resources

a. Retreats for interprofessional health professionals
b. Group work
c. Case studies
d. Reading material
e. Developing continuing professional development paths.

5. Formative assessment

a. Reflective Diary
b. Assignment on assessment of the setting discussed, either individual or as a group, describing the assessment process and the recommendations.

6. References

a. Abela, J., Mallia, P.
b. End of Life Care. A care worker handbook. Morris, C., Collier, F. Hodder Education, 2016.
c. Intelligent Kindness. Reforming the culture of healthcare. Ballatt, J., Campling, P. Royal College of Psychiatry Publication (UK), 2013.

7. Further Reading

a. British GMC Guidelines on End of Life.
b. McCarthy, J. et al (eds), *End of Life Care: Ethics and Law*. 1st edition. Cork University Press, 2011.

8. Internet resources

a. Futile Treatment at the end of life: legal, policy, sociological and economic perspectives: https://www.qut.edu.au/research-all/research-projects/futile-treatment-at-the-end-of-life
b. Futility and the Law: Knowledge, Practice and Attitudes of doctors at the end of life: https://papers.ssrn.com/sol3/papers.cfm?abstract_id=2802399
c. Reasons doctors provide 'futile' treatment at the end of life. An Australian qualitative study: http://www.preventingoverdiagnosis.net/2016Presentations/Lindy_Willmott.pdf
d. The courts, futility and the ends of medicine: https://www.ncbi.nlm.nih.gov/pmc/articles/PMC3530837/

Module 3

1. Title: **MEDICAL AND ETHICAL ISSUES.**
2. Introduction

   The ethical issues at the end of life are closely tied to the practice of medicine and part of the decision making process. In this sense they should not be separated into simply a biological process and a social one. Just as the decision to provide treatment rests on a family history, a past medical history, and a social history (usually implying substance abuse, living conditions etc), the latter, at the EoL should include the social and religious attitudes towards death.

   This understanding however has been implemented from place to place, and even ward to ward, in a very heterogeneous way, usually with the physician, who has ultimate responsibility, taking the risk or otherwise of the decision. In some wards and systems, conversely coherent approaches have been introduced. We often find that the delivery of high quality care depends on good pain relief, decision about what the patient considers as extraordinary measure, agreement about futile treatment, a good palliative care plan, and what people consider a 'good death', usually considered as dying in one's sleep and pain free surrounded by family and hopefully perhaps in familiar surroundings. This is however not frequently the case and there are bound to be disagreements. Often words like extraordinary and futile may be confused, and pain relief may be seen as hastening death.

   This module addresses these issues for health professionals so as to attempt a homogenous understanding of definitions and decision making process in order that the team is able to provide a coherent approach to EoL.
3. Learning Outcomes

   a. To learn about the coordination process when death is imminent. (Ch4)
   b. To be able to define and understand the various understanding of the delivery of high quality care. (Ch5)
   c. To understand the concept of Futility and why it's implications are important
   d. To understand what is extraordinary care and by whom it is defined and decided upon
   e. To have a sound knowing of pain relief and be able to explain the concept of double effect and how hastening death is not seen as immoral when an proper standard of care is followed.

4. Teaching and learning resources

   a. Retreats for interprofessional health professionals
   b. Group work
   c. Case studies
   d. Reading material
   e. Developing continuing professional development paths.

5. Formative assessment

a. Reflective Diary
b. Assignment on assessment of the setting discussed, either individual or as a group, describing the assessment process and the recommendations.

6. References
7. Further Reading

a. Advance Care Planning in End of Life Care; Thomas, K, Lobo, B. Oxford University Press, 2011
b. End of Life Care. A care worker handbook. Morris, C., Collier, F. Hodder Education, 2016.
c. Intelligent Kindness. Reforming the culture of healthcare. Ballatt, J., Campling, P. Royal College of Psychiatry Publication (UK), 2013.

8. Internet resources

a. Ethical Aspects in End of Life, Isish College of General Practitioners: https://www.icgp.ie/assets/4/080C4527-CDAE-E342-D365991EEFC98B2B_document/Medico-legal.pdf
b. End of Lfie Care. The Hasting Centre: http://www.thehastingscenter.org/briefingbook/end-of-life-care/

Module 4

1. Title: **SOCIAL ISSUES**
2. Introduction

   The end of life can be challenging not only to the patient but especially to the family, not to mention the health care professionals in dealing with social and cultural issues. Patients have preferences and life goals – things they wish to accomplish. Some have religious beliefs which may need clarification with family and health professionals. Others may wish to die at home or in a hospice-like setting.

   It is important to recognise the imminence of death – recognising that the patient may die within the year, and, recognising that the patient will die within the next few days. The first is important to start having discussions with relatives and patients in order to understand the goals and plan ahead. Health professionals need to know in good time what the preferences towards extraordinary treatment of the patient are and indeed the latter has to understand issues such as extraordinary care, futile treatment, CPR, etc. These issues become especially important if the patient wishes to die at home, where less technical assistance may be available, and where cultural issues about dying are involved.
3. Learning Outcomes

   a. To be able to recognise the imminence of death within one year, and the imminence of death within a few days.
   b. To learn about the difference between hospital and home care and to have an appreciation of what studies show about the preferences on patients and how this can be tackled at an early stage.
   c. To have an understanding of the various cultural issues which health care professionals face when dealing with end of life. This includes also disposal of bodies and other rituals and an understanding of the religious aspects of the communities in the setting.
   d. To appreciate what is meant by a 'good death' and how this is applicable to patients; and to be able to recognise the dying phase and undertake a plan of action.
   e. To learn how to undertake a needs assessment and a plan of care, understanding what the priorities are taking into consideration faith, worries, restriction owing to culture, and life goals.
   f. To learn the importance of conversations with patients and families towards the end of life.

4. Teaching and learning resources

   a. Retreats for interprofessional health professionals
   b. Group work
   c. Case studies
   d. Reading material
   e. Developing continuing professional development paths.

5. Formative assessment
   a. Reflective Diary
   b. Assignment on assessment of the setting discussed, either individual or as a group, describing the assessment process and the recommendations.
6. References

   a. Hayes, A., Henry, C., Holloway, M., Lindsey, K., Sherwen, E., Smith, T. *Pathways through care at the end of life. A guide to patient-centred care.* Jessica Kingsley Publishers, ondon and Philadelphia, 2014
   b. Middleton, L., Chatterjee, J., Russell, S., Downs, M. *End of Life Care for People with Dementia. A person-centred approach.* University of Bradford 'Dementia Good Practice guides', Jessica Kingsley Publishers, ondon and Philadelphia, 2017
   c. Thomas, K., Lobo, B., (Eds.). *Advance Care Planning in End of Life Care*, Oxford University Press, Oxford, New York, 2011.

7. Further Reading
   a. CME Palliative medicine, Hicks., F. (ed) *Clinical Medicine* Vol. 10, No.3: 275-278. 2010.
8. Internet resources
   a. American Psychological Association. End of Life issues and Care: http://www.apa.org/topics/death/end-of-life.aspx
   b. MedLine Plus. End of life issues: https://medlineplus.gov/endoflifeissues.html
   c. National Association of Social Workers (USA). *End of Life Care*: http://www.socialworkers.org/practice/bereavement/updates/EndofLifeCare-PU0204.pdf

Module 5

1. Title: **SPIRITUALITY**
2. Introduction

   Spiritual care is often used synonymously with spiritual and existential care; it includes care which is both specifically religious and regard for the existential issues and concerns that a dying person may go through. On the verge of death a person may be confronted with great existential issues such as the meaning of the life lived, the loss of life and the relationship with the next-of-kin, about faith in God, and faith in life after death. A person also experiences a series of agonising losses; as a result of impairment of health a person may not continue to preserve social relations and activities which before could be done.

   Faith and religiousness are a significant aspect of many people's outlook on life. It is important to acknowledge this and not in any way diminish their outlook at these final stages as it can increase existential suffering. The scope of religious care is not to triumph over death but rather to acknowledge the impotence one feels and that this is outside the power vested in any human being. Religious care helps the dying person to recognize the limits of his or her own power and to come to terms that God is taking over.
3. Learning Outcomes
   a. To understand how patients can be helped from a theological point of view, appreciating how they may be comforted through their religion.
   b. To appreciate the psychological perspective that it may be fear of death, desperation, anger or difficult relations with next-of-kin which may need to be addressed.
   c. To realise that there may be an avoidance of contact with the dying person due to health professionals being trained to 'fix' things; and therefore to appreciate the importance to establish contact and be opportunistic to recognise points where they can offer some assistance, such as communion, or speaking with a spiritual person.
   d. To understand that it is primarily the doctor who speaks about the progression of the disease and hence the importance to build trust in order to foster confidence in order to encourage the patient not to postpone things and to plan ahead and indeed to find meaning.
4. Teaching and learning resources
   a. Retreats for interprofessional health professionals
   b. Group work
   c. Case studies
   d. Reading material
   e. Developing continuing professional development paths.
5. Formative assessment
   a. Reflective Diary

b. Assignment on assessment of the setting discussed, either individual or as a group, describing the assessment process and the recommendations.

6. References

a. 'Statement form the Danish council of ethics', Spiritual Care for the Dying {{419 The Danish Council of Ethics 2004;

7. Further Reading

There are many books on the topic of spirituality at the end of life and website like Amazon provide a good repertoire. However a good academic books is:

Henry S. Perkins *A Guide to Psychosocial and Spiritual Care at the End of Life*, Springer,

8. Internet resources

a. Spiritual Care at the End of Life: http://journals.rcni.com/doi/pdfplus/10.7748/ns2013.09.28.2.41.e7977
b. The essential elements of spirituality in end of life care: http:// www.professionalchaplains.org/files/publications/chaplaincy_today_online/volume_24/number_2/24_2scott.pdf
c. VanderWeele, T.J., Balboni, T.R., Koh, H.K., *Health and Spirituality*; http://jamanetwork.com/journals/jama/data/journals/jama/0/jama_vanderweele_2017_vp_170098.pdf
d. Nuffied Council – EoL document – section on Spirituality: (TO ADD)xxx

Module 6

1. Title: **COMMUNICATION AND CONFLICT RESOLUTION**
2. Introduction

Rationale: Conflict resolution is a multi-disciplinary, analytical, problem-solving approach to conflict that seeks to enable participants to work collaboratively towards its resolution.[17] Conflict in health care arises inevitably and they are a part of life. Of most concern are the intra- and inter-professional conflicts which often regard management of patient and disagreement about certain principles. More pertinent are conflict which arise between health care professionals and the patient or relatives regarding the treatment and management at the end of life.

Whilst these can be due to lack of proper training and protocol and indeed lack of public education about what is morally acceptable, this module tackles how one should approach conflicts and what can be done at an administrative level to introduce a pathway when this become necessary.

Conflicts arise mostly because relatives may feel that more can be done. It is often a case that there has not been enough communication beforehand either that their relative is dying or that the management may be shifting towards a more palliate approach and not enough had been communicated in this regard. This has to be acknowledged and again is treated in different modules. Nevertheless, even with proper structure conflicts will arise and often this applies to people wanting futile or extraordinary treatment to be given whilst health professionals feel that this may be harmful to the patient and increase discomfort or agony.

Whilst there are various models of conflict resolution there are many things in common and health care approaches are discussed here emphasising the contextual and local health priorities.

3. Learning Outcomes

   a. To be able to define conflict resolution, its inevitability and which conflicts can be eliminated, minimised or at least managed.
   b. To identify the key persons/professionals involved and understand their perceptions and perspectives.
   c. To learn how to analyse conflict and to distinguish and be able to explain the difference between conflicts and disputes.
   d. To learn about mediation and the conflict resolution process
   e. To learn about the communication skills necessary for conflict resolution and to plan and prepare for the process, including assessing whether there are communication skills courses available and whether any pathways exist in the work place of the participant.
   f. To identify and learn what to do when things go wrong
   g. To understand the conflict resolution process within the remits of the Law, and Ethics

---

[17] Tillett, G., *Resoliving Conflict. A Practical Approach*. Oxford University Press, 2002, p1.

4. Teaching and learning resources
   a. Work based experience
      i. Participants are encouraged to bring cases and describe them in detail from their own work experience. These will be discussed to see whether and how a conflict resolution process could have helped or changed the outcome.
   b. Other learning opportunities
      i. Retreats
      ii. Workshops
      iii. Seminars
      iv. CPD
5. Formative Assessment
   a. Reflective diary
   b. Case discussions
   c. Feedback on how the participant thinks that this modules can change his or her practice and what pathways may be necessary to work towards.
6. References

   a. Tillett, G., *Resolving Conflict. A Practical Approach*, Oxford University Press, 1999.

7. Further reading

   a. Debono, E. *Conflicts. A Better way to resolve them.* Penguin Books, Harmsworth, UK, 1985.
   b. Lloyd, M., Bor, R. *Communication skills for Medicine*, Churchill Livinston/Elsevier, UK, 2009.
   c. Burnard, P., *Counselling skills for Health Professionals,* Stanley Thorns Publishers Ltd., UK, 1999.
   d. Tillett, G., *Resoliving Conflict. A Practical Approach.* Oxford University Press, 2002
   e. Lashley, J., *Confidence in Conflict for Health Care Profesionnals.* Turths Publishing, Milwaukee, USA. 2016

8. Internet resource(s):
   a. 'new approach to end of life care replaces axed Liverpool Care Pathway': https://www.nursingtimes.net/clinical-archive/end-of-life-and-palliative-care/new-approach-to-end-of-life-care-replaces-axed-liverpool-pathway/5072421.article
   b. End of Life care pathways for the dying: http://www.cochrane.org/CD008006/SYMPT_end-life-care-pathways-dying

c. New guidelines on end of life care published by NICE: http://www.nhs.uk/news/2015/12December/Pages/New-guidelines-on-end-of-life-care-published-by-NICE.aspx
d. Conflict Resolution in End of Life Care Settings (CRELS): https://stgrenal.org.au/sites/default/files/upload/Renal_supportive_care/conflict-resolution.pdf
e. Conflict resolutions in end of life treatment decisions: a rapid review: http://www.health.nsw.gov.au/research/Documents/14-conflict-resolution-end-of-life.pdf
f. Managing conflict at End of life (NEJM): http://www.nejm.org/doi/full/10.1056/NEJMp058104#t=article
g. Handing conflict in end of life care (JAMA): http://jamanetwork.com/journals/jama/article-abstract/1030825
h. Communication with patients and families: http://www.cpd.utoronto.ca/endoflife/Modules/COMMUNICATIONS%20MODULE.pdf
i. RCN end of life care – communication: http://rcnendoflife.org.uk/communication/

Module 7

1. Title: **THINKING ABOUT AND FORMULATING PATHWAYS**
2. Introduction

All systems have their strengths and weakness. This is inevitable and there should be timely assessments to assess efficiency, effectiveness and health patient experience. This is especially so in end of life care. Inevitably as well there can be conflict both intra-professionally and inter-professionally. The immense amount of literature, including academic articles, and book publications on the topic show that in many countries the end of life process is being questioned. Has end of life become too technical and medicalised? Do people, especially relatives, expect more out of a health care setting? Do people know about their own religious affiliation and what it may say about end of life care?

Health care professionals are numerous and strategically placed to assess patient experience and needs. They also know the inherent problems in the system, which they may attribute to their own profession or to another (nurses may blame doctors, doctors may blame administration, etc). The truth is that this blame-game is often wrong and that there are many facets to each problem, not least because something which used to work very well a decade before, and which has not been revised for changes occurring continuously, may not be working well now if it has not been periodically assessed.

The module bring together professionals working in end of life, or at least who experience end of life in their ward, to discuss the issues by bringing out worries and concerns and together try to assess what protocols are in place or need to be in place and to work together as a team to effect change. This 'medical leadership' involves learning how to make objective assessments, create a plan, or pathway, and bring this into effect. These pathways may involve either continuing professional development plans, or they may need the 'muscle' of the administration of the hospital. Conversely the problem may be regional or in the whole country (as was the case in the UK with the Liverpool Care Pathway, which from a good intention lacked certain training to make it useful. It was efficient but not effective. Therefore participants learn to identify whether one needs pathways even outside their setting, such as unions, associations, and indeed political.

Again some limitations may be due to lack of understand of the public about systems which may involve, for example, social teaching on end of life. In this case religious institutions may be the pathway to follow and which can work together with health professionals to promote media and talk to the public. Religious institutions may be known for defending principles of life which often lead to negative talk such as that of opposing euthanasia. But they may be very effective in relating what is actually *not* euthanasia and that which is licit, such as giving pain relief even if this may hasten death, once the intention is solely to relieve pain, or withdrawing/withholding disproportionate treatment.

The aim of the module is therefore twofold: the first is the help professionals identify and develops pathways to change for better patient experience; the second is to propose a remedy to the often helplessness that the same professionals field in view of negative experiences or lack of communication or proper protocol. In this way professionals become the medium for a change which is not based on subjective outside observation only but also on experience and objective assessment and use of tools to effect change.

3. Learning Outcomes

   a. To be able to think about the weakness in one's system, assess and formulate a pathway towards addressing the issues.
   b. To consider the various opportunities towards dealing with pathways, including political, social (including Patient Organisations, Religious institutions, etc), and administrative (Hospital, departments etc.)
   c. To be able to approach the various categories listed in b.
   d. To learn how to make objective assessments
   e. To learn how to think about and formulate an Advanced Care Plan.

4. Teaching and learning resources

   a. Retreats for interprofessional health professionals
   b. Workshops
   c. Reading material
   d. Developing continuing professional development paths.

5. Formative assessment

   a. Reflective Diary
   b. Work group presentation on an identified issue

6. References

   a. Saunders, J., (TO ADD)

7. Further Reading

   a. Hayes, et al., *Pathways through care at the end of life*, Jessica Kingsley Publishers, London and Philadelphia, 2014.
   b. CME Palliative Medicine, Hicks, F. (ed), in *Clinical Medicine* 2010, Vol 10, No 3: 275-8.

8. Internet resources

   a. Developing Pathways – NHS Network: https://www.networks.nhs.uk/nhs-networks/smart-guides/documents/Developing%20pathways%20-%20using%20patient%20and%20carer%20experiences.pdf
   b. What is a clinical pathway? Developing a definition to inform the debate: https://www.ncbi.nlm.nih.gov/pmc/articles/PMC2893088/
   c. Mapping out the patient's journey: experiences of developing pathways of care: https://www.ncbi.nlm.nih.gov/pmc/articles/PMC2893088/
   d. Developing pathways is a team effort: https://www.ahcmedia.com/articles/134556-developing-pathways-should-be-a-team-effort-experts-say

Resources:

Advance Care Planning in End of Life Care; Thomas, K, Lobo, B. Oxford University Press, 2011
Being Mortal. Illness, Mediine and what Matters in the End. Gawande, A., Wellcome Collection, Profile Books, 2015.
Biopsychosocial Medicine
Communication Skills for Medicine. Lloyd, M., Bor, R. Churchill Livingston. Elsevier, 2009.
Educating the Future GP. The Course Organiser's handbook. 2nd ed. McEvoy, P., Radcliff Medical Press, 1998.
End of Life Care for People with Dementia. A person-centred approach. Middleton-Green, L., et al. Jessica Kingsley Publishers, 2017.
End of Life Care. A care worker handbook. Morris, C., Collier, F. Hodder Education, 2016.
Extreme Measures. Finding a better path to the end of life. Nutik Zitter, J., Avery, New York, 2017.
Intelligent Kindness. Reforming the culture of healthcare. Ballatt, J., Campling, P. Royal College of Psychiatry Publication (UK), 2013.
Medical Decision Making. A physician's guide. Schwartz, A., Bergus, G. Cambridge Medicine, Cambridge University Press, Cambridge, New York, 2008.
Medical Futility. A Cross-national Study. Bagheri, A., (ed), Imperial College Press, 2013.
Oxford Textbook of Palliative Care to add
Palliative Care Nursing. Principles and Evidence for Practice. Payne, S., Seymour, J., Ingleton, C. McGraw Hill, Open University Press, 2008.
Pathways through care at the end of life. A guide to patient-centred care; Hayes, A. et al., Jessica Kingsley Publishers, 2014.
Psychology and Sociology applied to illness
Resolving Conflict. A Practical Approach. Tillett, G., Oxford University Press, 2002
The Inner Consultation, Neighbour, R., Petroc Press, 2002
The Philosophy of Palliative care. Critique and Construction. Randall, F., Downie, R. Oxford University Press, 2006.
The Way We Die Now. O'Moahony, S, Head of Zeus Ltd., UK, 2016

The Curriculum was developed as part of the European Union Project Erasmus+ EndCare project on Harmonisation of good practice at the end of life.

The partners were:

The Bioethics Research Programme of the University of Malta
The Centre for Ethics of the Dublin City University, Ireland
The Universita' degli studi dell'Aquila, Italy

It was also developed with the help of experts from the United Kingdom, France, Belgium, The faculties of Laws, Medicine & Surgery, and Theology of the University of Malta, Iran, UNESCO, The Pontifical Academy for Life, and Duquesne University, Pennsylvania, USA.

The manufacturer's authorised representative in the EU is Springer Nature Customer Service Centre GmbH, Europaplatz 3, 69115 Heidelberg, Germany. If you have any concerns regarding our products, please contact ProductSafety@springernature.com

Printed and bound by CPI Group (UK) Ltd, Croydon, CR0 4YY
28/09/2026
02224092-0001